Child Care & Development

Revision Exercises

Pamela Minett

Hodder Arnold

A MEMBER OF THE HODDER HEADLINE GROUP

Orders: please contact Bookpoint Ltd, 130 Milton Park, Abingdon,
Oxon OX14 4SB. Telephone: +44 (0)1235 827720. Fax: +44 (0)1235 400454.
Lines are open from 9.00—6.00, Monday to Saturday, with a 24-hour
message-answering service.
You can also order through our website www.hodderheadline.co.uk.

British Library Cataloguing in Publication Data
A catalogue record for this title is available from the British Library

ISBN-10: 0 340 88916 0
ISBN-13: 978 0 340 88916 9

First published 2005
Impression number   10 9 8 7 6 5 4 3 2 1
Year   2007 2006 2005

Typeset by Dorchester Typesetting Group Limited
Printed in Great Britain for Hodder & Stoughton Educational, a division of
Hodder Headline, 338 Euston Road, London NW1 3BH by CPI, Bath.

Child Care
& Development

sion

ises

USING THIS BOOK

These *Revision Exercises* reinforce the subject matter contained in the textbook *Child Care & Development* (ISBN 0 340 88915 2). They also cover the core material in most courses with a child care or child development element, for example GCSE Home Economics: Child Development, the CACHE Foundation Award in Caring for Children, CACHE Level 2 Certificate in Child Care and Education, SVQ and NVQ Level 2 in Early Years Care and Education, and a wide range of health and social care courses.

Although written to accompany the textbook, this book has been compiled as a totally separate book and can stand alone as a student's revision guide in reinforcing other textbooks and resource materials that are being used. Each exercise consists of two pages, one page contains questions, and, overleaf, the second page contains the answers in sentence form, with explanations where appropriate. This format enables students to work independently of the teacher, marking their own work, identifying areas of weakness, revising and then re-testing themselves.

Child Care & Development: Revision Exercises is an invaluable resource, not only as a revision aid, but also to students who have missed part of a course through illness, late starting, lack of time or other reasons.

Pamela Minett

CONTENTS

SECTION 1 THE FAMILY AND HOME

CONTENTS

1   Match up children's needs with the reason for them

Children need:	Reason:
i food and drink	to keep them safe
ii love and companionship	to prepare them for adult life
iii protection and support	so that they are socially acceptable
iv education and training	so they can learn how to speak
v people who talk to them	being too cold or over-heated can kill
vi boundaries for behaviour	to make them feel loved and wanted
vii enough warmth and clothing	for growth and energy

---

2   Use these words to complete the sentences below: **one-parent   extended   step   nuclear**

Sarah lived with her parents and brother and was part of a .... family. This became

an .... family when her grandparents came to live with them. Sarah married and

had three children; they became a .... family when her husband left the family

home. When Sarah married again they became a .... family.

---

3 Families caring for children not related to
them are:
  A shared-care families
  B extended families
  C foster families
  D nuclear families

4 Co-habiting means:
  A married couples living together
  B married couples living apart
  C unmarried couples not living together
  D any couple living together

Households in Gt Britain, 2002 (*Source: General Household Survey*)

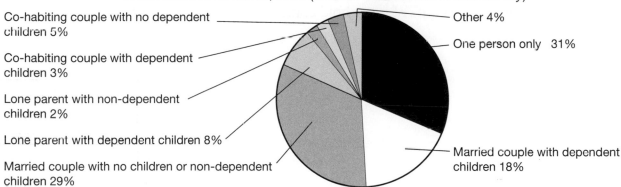

Co-habiting couple with no dependent children 5%

Co-habiting couple with dependent children 3%

Lone parent with non-dependent children 2%

Lone parent with dependent children 8%

Married couple with no children or non-dependent children 29%

Other 4%

One person only   31%

Married couple with dependent children 18%

---

5 Use the pie chart to complete the percentages of households with dependent children in 2002

		1996	2002
i	married couples with dependent children	23%	....
ii	co-habiting couples with dependent children	3%	....
iii	lone parent with dependent children	7%	....
iv	total households with dependent children	33%	....

6 Between 1996 and 2002, did the number of households with children increase or decrease?

....

7 In 2002, which type of household was the most common? ....

1 Children need:
   i   food and drink **for growth and energy**
   ii   enough warmth and clothing because **being too cold or over-heated can kill**
   iii love and companionship **to make them feel loved and wanted**
   iv   protection and support **to keep them safe**
   v   education and training **to prepare them for adult life**
   vi   people who talk to them **so they can learn how to speak**
   vii boundaries for behaviour **so that they are socially acceptable.**

2 Sarah lived with her parents and brother and was part of a **nuclear** family. This became an **extended** family when her grandparents came to live with them. Sarah married and had three children; they became a **lone-parent** family when her husband left the family home. When Sarah married again they became a **step**-family.

3 Families caring for children not related to them are **foster families**.

4 Co-habiting means **any couple living together**.

5
Households by family type	1996	2002
i married couples with dependent children	23%	**18%**
ii co-habiting couples with dependent children	3%	**3%**
iii lone parent with dependent children	7%	**8%**
iv total households with dependent children	<u>33%</u>	<u>**29%**</u>

6 Comparing 1996 and 2002, the number of households with children **decreased**.

7 In 2002, the most common type of household contained **one person only**.

Total number of marks	19
First time score	....
Score after revision	....

During the last century, there were many changes to **family** life in Britain.

Small families became more common. **Divorce** became easier.

Many **women** with **dependent** children also had **jobs** outside the **home**.

Many **fathers** began to help with the day-to-day care of their **children**.

Women got the **vote**, and the same **education** and **career** prospects as men.

Working hours became shorter, and **holidays** longer.

The general **standard** of living greatly **improved**, and many people owned **cars**.

Every family expected to have its own home, piped **water** supply, **electricity** and **television**.

Complete this wordsearch by finding all the words above which are in **bold** type. The words can be horizontal, vertical or diagonal, forwards or backwards,

F	A	T	H	E	R	S	E	X	A	D	H	G	N	O	I
Y	B	F	O	U	B	B	A	I	R	S	S	O	R	T	M
N	S	I	L	K	O	O	P	A	E	M	D	E	M	A	P
E	P	M	I	N	E	J	D	E	R	A	W	A	T	E	R
N	N	O	D	T	T	N	E	S	A	K	O	R	U	Q	O
C	T	R	A	D	A	N	G	T	C	A	R	E	E	R	V
I	V	E	Y	T	H	T	D	H	O	L	K	I	W	T	E
R	F	O	S	T	E	L	E	V	I	S	I	O	N	P	D
L	S	O	P	S	A	E	P	R	O	L	N	W	O	T	T
Y	L	I	M	A	F	R	E	D	R	E	G	Y	I	R	D
C	E	A	W	E	X	G	N	B	L	E	P	O	T	Y	I
S	L	N	C	H	I	L	D	R	E	N	B	L	A	E	V
L	P	W	E	U	M	R	E	A	N	P	Q	J	C	O	O
S	C	T	W	O	M	E	N	I	C	A	R	S	U	M	R
D	O	E	W	V	E	N	T	O	P	W	B	L	D	O	C
V	U	N	H	T	Y	T	I	C	I	R	T	C	E	L	E

FAMILY

SMALL

DIVORCE

WOMEN

DEPENDENT

JOBS

HOME

FATHERS

CHILDREN

VOTE

EDUCATION

CAREER

WORKING

HOLIDAYS

STANDARD

IMPROVED

CARS

WATER

ELECTRICITY

TELEVISION

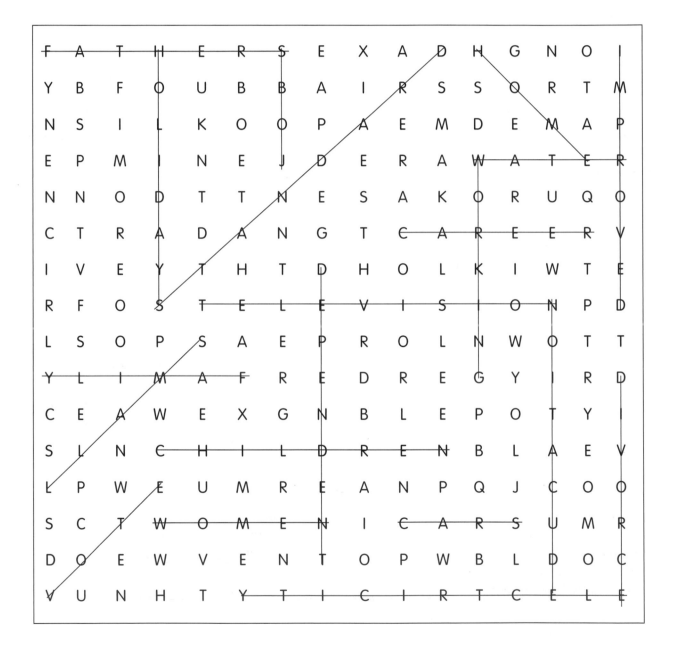

Total number of marks	20
First time score	....
Score after revision	....

1 Match up the statements to show some of the ways in which families vary:

i	The size of the family	healthy to unhealthy
ii	The ages of family members	strong belief to no belief
iii	Where the family lives	the same country to different countries
iv	Financial status	small to large
v	Health	urban (towns, cities) to rural (country)
vi	Country of origin	very young to very old
vii	Religious belief	rich to poor

2 Match up the statements to show how feelings of family members towards each other can vary:

i	From care	to fear
ii	From respect	to hate
iii	From love	to indifference
iv	From trust	to contempt

3 Use the words below to complete the sentences showing how attitudes of parents can vary:

no   **reasonably**   **unwanted**   **moderate**   **tolerated**   **neglect**

i   Children may be wanted by their parents or __ __ __ __ __ __ __ __ __ or

__ __ __ __ __ __ __ __ .

ii   Parents may overindulge their children or act __ __ __ __ __ __ __ __ __ __ or

__ __ __ __ __ __ __ them.

iii Parents may enforce strict discipline or __ __ __ __ __ __ __ __ discipline or __ __
discipline.

4 Ethnic groups are:
   A groups of people who come from different parts of the world
   B groups of people who follow the same religions
   C people of a mixture of nationalities
   D groups of people who speak different languages

5 Culture means:
   A living in a different society
   B having a different religion
   C the way of life of a group of people
   D coming from a different country

6 Multicultural means:
   A a person who speaks several languages
   B people with differing religions
   C human behaviour which has been learnt
   D people of different ethnic groups co-existing together

7 Religion
   A influences cultural life
   B has no effect on cultural life
   C has little effect on cultural life
   D has total effect on cultural life

1 Ways in which families vary:
  i   The size of the family – **small to large**
  ii   The ages of family members – **very young to very old**
  iii Where the family lives – **urban (towns, cities) to rural (country)**
  iv   Financial status – **rich to poor**
  v   Health – **healthy to unhealthy**
  vi   Country of origin – **the same country to different countries**
  vii Religious belief – **strong belief to no belief**

2 Feelings of family members towards each other vary:
  i   From care **to indifference**
  ii   From respect **to contempt**
  iii From love **to hate**
  iv   From trust **to fear**

3 Varying attitudes of parents to their children:
  i   Children may be wanted by their parents or **tolerated** or **unwanted**.   (2 marks)
  ii   Parents may over-indulge their children or act **reasonably** or **neglect** them.   (2 marks)
  iii Parents may enforce strict discipline or **moderate** discipline or **no** discipline. (2 marks)

4 Ethnic groups are **groups of people who come different parts of the world** and have their own racial or cultural background.

5 Culture means **the way of life of a group of people**, including their language, customs, values, beliefs and arts.

6 Multicultural means **people of different ethnic groups co-existing together**.

7 Religion **influences cultural life**.

Total number of marks	21
First time score	....
Score after revision	....

1 Match each type of development with its description:

i	Physical development	learning to control feelings
ii	Language development	learning to interact with people
iii	Social development	development of thinking and understanding
iv	Emotional development	development of the body
v	Intellectual (cognitive) development	learning to talk

1

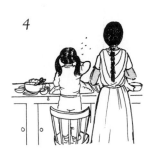

2

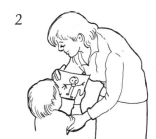

3

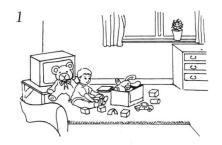

4

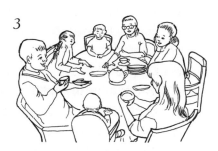

5

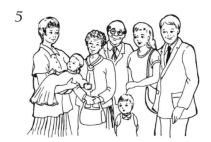

6

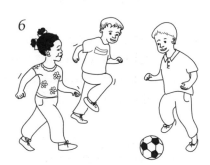

2 Of drawings 1–6 which provides an opportunity for a child to:

i	feel useful	....	vii	learn to draw	....
ii	play with others	....	viii	play outside	....
iii	play alone	....	ix	play inside	....
iv	be praised	....	x	talk with her mum	....
v	enjoy a family meal	....	xi	talk with his mum	....
vi	exercise	....	xii	meet other adults	.... and ....

3 Television is beneficial:
   A when it is on all the time
   B because it teaches children to talk
   C because children understand what they see
   D when adults watch with children and talk about what is seen

4 Television is harmful:
   A when it is on all the time
   B because it does not teach children to talk
   C because children understand what they see
   D when adults watch with children and talk about what is seen

1 i Physical development – **development of the body**
  ii Language development – **learning to talk**
  iii Social development – **learning to interact with people**
  iv Emotional development – **learning to control feelings**
  v Intellectual (cognitive) development – **development of thinking and understanding**

2 i feel useful   4
  ii play with others   6
  iii play alone   1
  iv be praised   2
  v enjoy a family meal   3
  vi exercise   6
  vii learn to draw   2
  viii play outside   6
  ix play inside   1
  x talk with her mum   4
  xi talk with his mum   2
  xii meet other adults   3 and 5

3 Television is beneficial **when adults watch with children and talk about what is seen**.

4 Television is harmful **when it is on all the time**.

Total number of marks	19
First time score	....
Score after revision	....

1 Use these words to complete the suggestions for parents below:

communicate   over-fussy   punishment   relationship   talk   security   understand

i   Love and cuddle your baby to give the baby the _ _ _ _ _ _ _ _ of feeling wanted.

ii   Speak to your baby so your baby can learn how to _ _ _ _ .

iii   Listen to your baby so you will learn how to _ _ _ _ _ _ _ _ _ _ _ with each other.

iv   Play with your baby to enable a closer _ _ _ _ _ _ _ _ _ _ _ _ to develop between you.

v   Keep your baby clean but do not be _ _ _ _ _ – _ _ _ _ _ .

vi   Be firm with your baby when your baby is old enough to _ _ _ _ _ _ _ _ _ _ what is wanted.

vii   Praise is more effective than _ _ _ _ _ _ _ _ _ _ in the training of children.

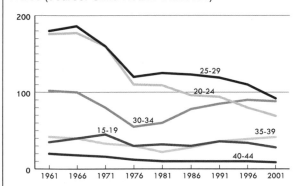

Live births per 1000 women by age group in England and Wales (*Source: Child Health Statistics*)

2 Which age group had the:

i   highest number of births? ....

ii   lowest number of births? ....

3 Which age group has shown the steepest decline in births since 1961? ....

4 Which two age groups had similar numbers of births in 1966 and 1991?

.... and ....

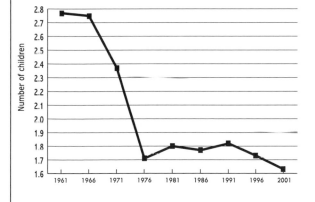

Number of children born for each woman in England and Wales (*Source: Population Trends*)

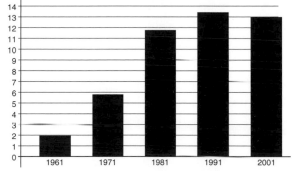

Divorces per 1000 married women in England and Wales (*Source: Child Health Statistics*)

5 During which 5 years did the number of children per woman:

i   fall below 2 per woman? .... and ....

ii   fall to its lowest level?   .... and ....

6 Did it take about 25, 35, 45 or 55 years for the number of children per woman to fall from over 2.7 to under 1.7? ....

7 The divorce rate per thousand married women in 1961 was ....

8 How many more women, per thousand, divorced in 2001 than in 1961? ....

9 In which year was the divorce rate for women at its highest? ....

1 **Suggestions for parents:**
    i   Love and cuddle your baby to give the baby the **security** of feeling wanted.
    ii   Speak to your baby so your baby can learn how to **talk**.
    iii Listen to your baby so you will learn how to **communicate** with each other.
    iv Play with your baby to enable a closer **relationship** to develop between you.
    v   Keep your baby clean but do not be **over-fussy**.
    vi Be firm with your baby when your baby is old enough to **understand** what is wanted.
    vii Praise is more effective than **punishment** in the training of children.

2   i   The **25–29** age group had the highest number of births.
     ii   The **40–44** age group had the lowest number of births.

3 The **20–24** age group has shown the steepest decline in births since 1961. In 1961 there were more than 170 births per thousand women; by 2001 the number had declined to about 70.

4 The **15–19** and **35–39** age groups had similar numbers of births in 1966 and 1991.

5   i   The number of children per woman fell below 2 between **1971** and **1976**.
     ii   The number of children per woman fell to its lowest level between **1996** and **2001**.

6 It took about **35** years for the number of children per woman to fall from over 2.7 to under 1.7.

7 The divorce rate per thousand married women in 1961 was **2**.

8 **11** more women, per thousand, divorced in 2001 than in 1961.

9 The divorce rate for women was at its highest in **1991**.

Total number of marks	17
First time score	....
Score after revision	....

1 Draw lines to match each method of contraception with its appropriate comment:

Method of contraception   **Comment**
i   abstaining (saying 'No' to intercourse)   placed over the cervix
ii   vasectomy   depend on knowledge of the menstrual cycle
iii contraceptive pills   very unreliable
iv   intrauterine system (IUS or the coil)   it is 100% safe
v   cap   contain hormones
vi   condom   placed over the penis
vii withdrawal   placed in the womb
viii natural methods   male sterilisation

2 Name the two methods of contraception above that help to avoid sexually transmitted diseases:

i   ....

ii   ....

3 Apart from abstaining, name the three methods above which do not require medical advice:

i   ....

ii   ....

iii ....

4 Sexual intercourse can result in pregnancy when it takes place:

☐ for the first time

☐ during a period

☐ when breast-feeding

☐ using the withdrawal method

5 Emergency contraception to prevent an unwanted pregnancy must occur within
  A a few days
  B the first week
  C the first two weeks
  D a month

6 Sexually transmitted infections are mainly:
  A air-borne diseases
  B diseases of the sex organs
  C caught by kissing
  D caught from coffee cups

7 Which is *not* a sexually transmitted disease?
  A HIV
  B chlamydia
  C tuberculosis
  D gonorrhoea

8 HIV is a:
  A protozoan
  B bacterium
  C microscopic fungus
  D virus

9 HIV is not caught from
  A infected blood
  B infected semen
  C infected vaginal fluid
  D dirty lavatory seats

10 Which sexually transmitted diseases can cause infertility in women?
  A gonorrhoea and chlamydia
  B chlamydia and thrush
  C thrush and genital warts
  D genital warts and gonorrhoea

1 i   abstaining (saying 'No' to intercourse) – **is 100% safe**
   ii   vasectomy – **male sterilisation**
   iii contraceptive pills – **contain hormones**
   iv   intrauterine system – **placed in the womb**
   v   cap – **placed over the cervix**
   vi   condom – **placed over the penis**
   vii withdrawal – **very unreliable**
   viii natural methods – **depend on knowledge of the menstrual cycle**

2 Two methods of contraception that help to avoid sexually transmitted diseases are:
   i   **abstaining (saying 'No' to intercourse)**
   ii   using **condoms**

3 Three methods of contraception that do not require medical advice are:
   i   **condoms**
   ii   **withdrawal**
   iii **natural methods** (these do not require medical advice, but instruction from a family
        planning clinic is advisable).

4 Pregnancy can result when sexual intercourse takes place:

   ☑ **for the first time**

   ☑ **during a period**

   ☑ **when breast-feeding**

   ☑ **using the withdrawal method** (sperm can swim)

5 Emergency contraception to prevent an unwanted pregnancy must occur within **the few
   days** following unprotected intercourse. Emergency contraceptive pills must be taken
   within three days, or a IUS coil fitted within five days.

6 Sexually transmitted infections are mainly **diseases of the sex organs**. An exception is HIV
   which, although it can be transmitted sexually, is a disease of the immune system.

7 **Tuberculosis** is not a sexually transmitted disease.

8 HIV is a **virus**. HIV stands for human immunodeficiency virus.

9 HIV is not caught from **dirty lavatory seats**.

10 The sexually transmitted diseases **gonorrhoea and chlamydia** can cause infertility in
   women.

Total number of marks	23
First time score	....
Score after revision	....

SECTION 2 BECOMING A PARENT

CONTENTS

1 The stage of development during which the sex organs mature is called _ _ _ _ _ _ _ _ _ .

2 Name three changes to the male body during puberty:

i ....

ii ....

iii ....

3 Use these terms to label the diagram below (hint: the number of dashes in each label equals the number of letters in each answer):

bladder	penis	scrotum	urethra
epididymis	prostate gland	testis	vas deferens
foreskin	seminal vesicle		

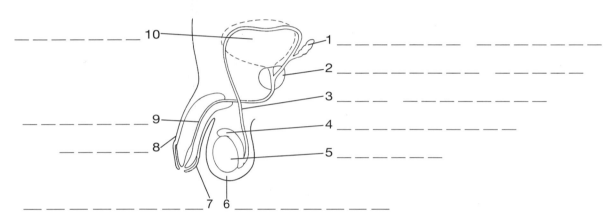

Side view of the male reproductive system

4 Use the terms above to answer the following questions:

i Where are sperm produced? ....

ii Where are sperm stored? ....

iii Name the bag containing the testicles: ....

iv Which part is also called the 'sperm tube'? ....

v Which part covers the tip of the penis? ....

vi Which part is removed in circumcision? ....

vii Which tube carries both semen and urine? ....

viii Which part is used for placing semen in the vagina of a female? ....

5 Semen contains:
  A sperm
  B sperm and fluid from the seminal vesicles
  C sperm and fluid from the prostate gland
  D sperm and fluid from the seminal vesicles and prostate gland

6 An ejaculate of semen normally contains:
  A hundreds of sperm
  B thousands of sperm
  C a million sperm
  D many millions of sperm

1 i The stage of development during which the sex organs mature is called **puberty**.

ii The testes produce the male hormone **testosterone**.

2 These changes happen to the male body during puberty:

shoulders broaden / male sex hormones are produced / testosterone is produced / sperm is produced / muscles develop / hair grows on the face (beard) / hair grows in the armpits / pubic hair grows / voice deepens

(3 marks)

3 1 **seminal vesicle**

2 **prostate gland**

3 **vas deferens**

4 **epididymis**

5 **testis**

6 **scrotum**

7 **foreskin**

8 **penis**

9 **urethra**

10 **bladder**

4 i Sperm are produced in the **testes** (singular: **testis**).

ii Sperm are stored in the **epididymis**.

iii The **scrotum** contains the testicles. Each testicle consists of testis and epididymis.

vi The sperm tube is also called the **vas deferens**.

v The tip of the penis is covered by the **foreskin**.

vi The **foreskin** is removed in circumcision.

vii The **urethra** carries both semen and urine.

viii The **penis** is used for placing semen in the vagina of a female.

5 Semen contains **sperm and fluid from the seminal vesicles and prostate gland.**

6 An ejaculate of semen normally contains **many millions of sperm.**

Total number of marks	25
First time score	....
Score after revision	....

1 Name three changes to the female body during puberty:

i   ....

ii ....

iii ....

2 Use the terms below to label parts 1–10 of the diagram below (hint: the number of dashes in each label equals the number of letters in each answer):

cervix	uterus	Fallopian tube	urethra	anus
ovary	vagina	funnel	uterus lining	bladder

Side view of the female reproductive system

3   Which of the parts in Question 2

i   produces eggs? ....

ii   is also called 'egg tube' or 'oviduct'?..

iii is where sperm are deposited during intercourse? ....

iv   catches the egg when it is released from the ovary? ....

v   is the technical name for the womb?

vi   is the technical name for the 'neck of the womb'?...

vii produces cervical mucus?..

viii is where a baby develops? ....

ix   consists of a large amount of muscle tissue? ....

x   is shed during menstruation? ....

4 The technical name for an egg is:
  A ovum
  B embyro
  C zygote
  D ova

5 Fertilisation takes place in:
  A a Fallopian tube
  B an ovary
  C the uterus
  D the vagina

1   These changes happen to the female body during puberty:
female sex hormones are produced / oestrogen is produced / periods start / hair grows in armpits / pubic hair grows / hips broaden / ovaries produce eggs / breasts develop

(3 marks)

2   1 **funnel**
2 **ovary**
3 **uterus**
4 **cervix**
5 **vagina**
6 **anus**
7 **urethra**
8 **bladder**
9 **uterus lining**
10 **Fallopian tube**

3   i   Eggs are produced in the **ovary**
ii   A **Fallopian tube** is also called an egg tube or oviduct
iii Sperm are deposited in the **vagina** during intercourse
iv   Eggs are caught in the **funnel**
v   The technical name for the womb is **uterus**
vi   The technical name for the neck of the womb is **cervix**
vii Cervical mucus is produced by the **cervix**
viii A baby develops in the **uterus**
ix   The **uterus** consists of muscle
x   The **uterus lining** is shed during menstruation

4   The technical name for an egg is **ovum**.

5   Fertilisation takes place in a **Fallopian tube**.

Total number of marks	25
First time score	....
Score after revision	....

1 Use the terms below to label the four phases A–D of the menstrual cycle
pre-menstrual phase
repair phase
receptive phase
menstruation

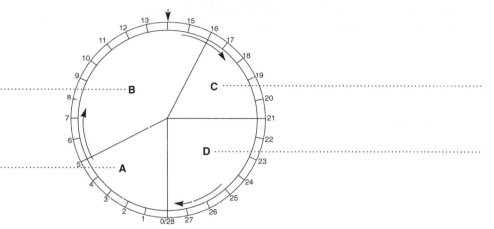

Diagram of a typical menstrual cycle

2 The purpose of the menstrual cycle is to:
  A renew the lining of the womb
  B prepare the uterus to receive a fertilised egg
  C prepare a place for fertilisation to take place
  D get rid of unwanted blood

3 The arrow at day 14 indicates:
  A fertilisation
  B ovulation
  C implantation
  D conception

4 Use the diagram of conception to help fill in the missing words in the text below:

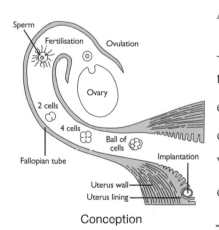

Conception

After _ _ _ _ _ _ _ _ _ _ , the egg moves into the

_ _ _ _ _ _ _ _ _ _ _ _ _ . If sexual intercourse has

taken place recently, many _ _ _ _ _ _ _ will surround the

egg. After being _ _ _ _ _ _ _ _ _ _ _ , the egg starts to

divide first into _ _ _ _ cells, then _ _ _ _ _ , and so on.

When it reaches the _ _ _ _ _ _ _ , it is a hollow _ _ _ _

of cells. About six days after fertilisation, it becomes

_ _ _ _ _ _ _ _ _ _ in the _ _ _ _ _ _ _

_ _ _ _ _ _ _ .

5 Which is the main male sex hormone?
  A progesterone
  B prolactin
  C oxytocin
  D testosterone

6 Which of these hormones is most important in maintaining pregnancy?
  A progesterone
  B prolactin
  C oxytocin
  D testosterone

7 Which hormone controls milk production?
  A progesterone
  B prolactin
  C oxytocin
  D testosterone

8 Which hormone stimulates the uterus to contract during childbirth?
  A progesterone
  B prolactin
  C oxytocin
  D testosterone

1   A   menstruation
       B   repair phase
       C   receptive phase
       D   pre-menstrual phase

2   The purpose of the menstrual cycle is to **prepare the uterus to receive a fertilised egg**.

3   The arrow at day 14 represents **ovulation**.

4   After **ovulation**, the egg moves into the **Fallopian tube**. If sexual intercourse has taken place recently, many **sperms** will surround the egg. After being **fertilised**, the egg starts to divide first into **two** cells, then **four**, and so on. When it reaches the **uterus**, it is a hollow **ball** of cells. About six days after fertilisation, it becomes **implanted** in the **uterus lining**.

5   **Testosterone** is the main male sex hormone.

6   **Progesterone** is the most important hormone in maintaining pregnancy.

7   Milk production is controlled by **prolactin**.

8   **Oxytocin** stimulates the uterus to contract during childbirth.

Total number of marks	20
First time score	....
Score after revision	....

1 Add these labels to the diagram of the foetus.
amnion
amniotic fluid
cervix
foetus
placenta
umbilical cord
uterus wall

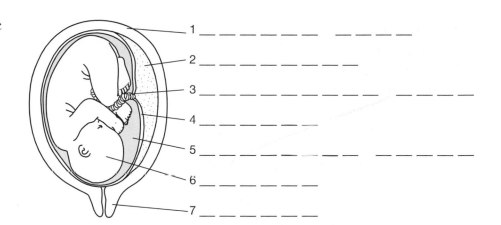

1 _ _ _ _ _ _ _ _ _ _

2 _ _ _ _ _ _ _ _

3 _ _ _ _ _ _ _ _ _ _ _ _ _

4 _ _ _ _ _ _

5 _ _ _ _ _ _ _ _ _ _ _ _ _ _ _

6 _ _ _ _ _ _ _

7 _ _ _ _ _ _

2 Give the number of the part in the diagram above which

i is a liquid ....

ii can grow to about 50 cm long ....

iii cushions the baby against shocks ....

iv is a ring of muscle ....

3 Use words from the diagram above to fill in the spaces.

Besides producing the embryo, the fertilised egg also gives rise to the _ _ _ _ _ _ _ _ _ ,

the _ _ _ _ _ _ _ _ _ _ _ _ _ _ and the _ _ _ _ _ _ _ . As the embryo

becomes more human-like it is called a _ _ _ _ _ _ _ .

4 The umbilical cord contains:
A blood vessels from the baby
B the mother's blood vessels
C blood vessels of both mother and baby
D no blood vessels

5 Which of these substances is able to cross the placenta from mother to baby?
A antibodies
B platelets
C white cells
D red cells

6 Which of these substances does **not** pass across the placenta from mother to baby?
A chemicals from smoke
B viruses
C alcohol
D white cells

7 Which of these substances crosses the placenta from baby to mother?
A carbon dioxide
B platelets
C white cells
D red cells

8 The placenta
A acts as a cushion for the baby
B digests food for the baby
C breathes for the baby
D supplies the baby with food and oxygen

9 An ectopic pregnancy occurs when an embryo
A produces a very large baby
B becomes inplanted outside the uterus
C divides to form twins
D becomes implanted inside the uterus

10 Pre-term babies are those born before
A 37 weeks
B 38 weeks
C 39 weeks
D 40 weeks

11 The rate at which miscarriages occur is estimated to be:
A 1 in every 2 pregnancies
B 1 in every 8 pregnancies
C 1 in every 40 pregnancies
D 1 in every 100 pregnancies

1   1   uterus wall
      2   placenta
      3   umbilical cord
      4   amnion
      5   amniotic fluid
      6   foetus
      7   cervix

2   i   part **5** is a liquid
      ii   part **3** can grow to about 50 cm long
      iii part **5** cushions the foetus against shocks
      iv part **7** is a ring of muscle

3 Besides producing the embryo, the fertilised egg also gives rise to the **placenta**, the **umbilical cord** and the **amnion**. As the embryo becomes more human-like it is called a **foetus**.

4 The umbilical cord contains **blood vessels** from the baby.

5 **Antibodies** cross the placenta from mother to baby.

6 **White cells** cannot cross the placenta from mother to baby.

7 **Carbon dioxide** crosses the placenta from baby to mother to be excreted.

8 The placenta **supplies the baby with food and oxygen**.

9 An ectopic pregnancy occurs when an embryo **becomes implanted outside the uterus**.

10 Pre-term babies are those born before **37 weeks**.

11 It is estimated that **1 in every 8** pregnancies ends in miscarriage, most occurring in the first three months.

Total number of marks	23
First time score	....
Score after revision	....

1 Pre-conception care applies to:
A women who are pregnant
B women who hope to become pregnant
C the unborn baby
D pre-term babies

2 Is folic acid
A vitamin E
B another name for vitamin C
C one of the B vitamins
D vitamin K?

3 Which of these foods contain folic acid?
A pickles and spices
B bread and green vegetables
C milk and milk products
D meat and fish

4 Folic acid is important before and during early pregnancy because it helps to prevent:
A Down's syndrome
B spina bifida
C cystic fibrosis
D cerebral palsy

5 The most reliable indication of pregnancy is:
A increased appetite
B morning sickness
C a missed period
D fainting

6 Pregnant women are advised to avoid:
A UHT milk
B pasteurised goats' milk
C unpasteurised milk
D sterilised milk

7 Which of the following should not be taken during pregnancy without first seeking a doctor's opinion?
A travel sickness pills
B antibiotics
C cough medicines
D all of the above

8 Which infectious disease can be dangerous to an unborn baby?
A rubella
B whooping cough
C mumps
D chicken pox

9 Toxoplasmosis can be caught from
A soft cheeses
B newborn lambs
C a cat's litter tray
D dogs' droppings

10 Chlamydiosis can be caught from
A soft cheeses
B newborn lambs
C a cat's litter tray
D dogs' droppings

11 Listeriosis can be caught from
A soft cheeses
B newborn lambs
C a cat's litter tray
D dogs' droppings

12 Compared with babies born to non-smoking mothers, babies born to smokers are, on average:
A smaller but just as healthy
B smaller and less healthy
C the same size but less healthy
D larger but less healthy

13 The chemical in smoke that is thought to affect a baby's growth is:
A carbon dioxide
B oxygen
C nitrogen
D carbon monoxide

14 To prevent smoke affecting their unborn babies' weight, pregnant women need to have given up smoking by the
A 2nd month of pregnancy
B 3rd month of preganancy
C 4th month of pregnancy
D 5th month of pregnancy

15 After they are born, which conditions are more likely to affect babies who regularly inhale people's smoke?
i bronchitis ☐
ii impetigo ☐
iii scabies ☐
iv pneumonia ☐
v tetanus ☐
vi cot death ☐

1 Pre-conception care applies to **women who hope to become pregnant**.

2 Folic acid is **one of the B vitamins**.

3 **Bread and green vegetables** contain folic acid.

4 Folic acid helps to prevent **spina bifida**.

5 The most reliable indication of pregnancy is **a missed period**.

6 Pregnant women are advised to avoid **unpasteurised milk**.

7 **None of the medicines** should be taken during pregnancy without a doctor's consent.

8 **Rubella** can be dangerous to an unborn baby in the first four months of pregnancy. The baby may be stillborn or born deaf, blind, have heart disease or a learning disability.

9 Toxoplasmosis can be caught from a cat's faeces in **a cat's litter tray**.

10 Chlamydiosis can be caught from **newborn lambs** and from sheep who have recently given birth.

11 Listeriosis can be caught from **soft cheeses** such as camembert and blue-veined cheese.

12 Babies born to mothers who smoke are, on average, **smaller and less healthy**.

13 **Carbon monoxide** is thought to affect a baby's growth.

14 To prevent smoke affecting their unborn babies' weight, pregnant women need to give up smoking by the **fourth month of pregnancy**.

15 Babies who regularly inhale other people's smoke are more likely to suffer from:
bronchitis
pneumonia
cot death.

Total number of marks	17
First time score	....
Score after revision	....

1 An expectant mother needs to eat:
   A enough for two
   B extra carbohydrates for energy
   C extra protein and fat for the baby
   D extra protein, vitamins and minerals

2 Nausea (feeling sick) during pregnancy can occur:
   A in the mornings
   B in the evenings
   C in the mornings and evenings
   D at any time

3 Heartburn is:
   A a burning sensation in the heart
   B indigestion
   C a burning sensation in the chest
   D an overactive heart

4 Hormones are substances which
   A help to regulate the way the body works
   B only become active during pregnancy
   C are similar to vitamins
   D are similar to minerals

---

5 Match each of these conditions associated with pregnancy with the appropriate advice:
   i   Pregnancy sickness   avoid standing for too long
   ii Heartburn   eat plenty of fruit, vegetables and fibre
   iii Constipation   usually disappears after the first three months
   iv Varicose veins   eat small meals and sleep propped up

---

6 Complete the crossword puzzle:

Across
1 They may share the same placenta (5)
4 Delivery (5)
7 Childbirth nurse (7)
8 Expected date of delivery (3)
9 Ovum (3)
10 Infants (6)
11 Toxoplasmosis can be caught from the faeces of these animals (4)
14 It is unusual for a pregnant woman to be given an X-_ _ _ (3)
15 Hepa _ _ _ _ (5)
16 Eggs (3)
18 Womb (6)

Down
1 Abdomen (5)
2 Intra-uterine device (3)
3 Related to chicken pox (8)
4 Born bottom first (6)
5 German measles (7)
6 Top part of the body (4)
9 Has 'gills' and a 'tail' (6)
12 Pregnancy _ _ _ _ _ are done on samples of urine (5)
13 Bigness or smallness (4)
17 N _ _ sea means feeling sick (2)

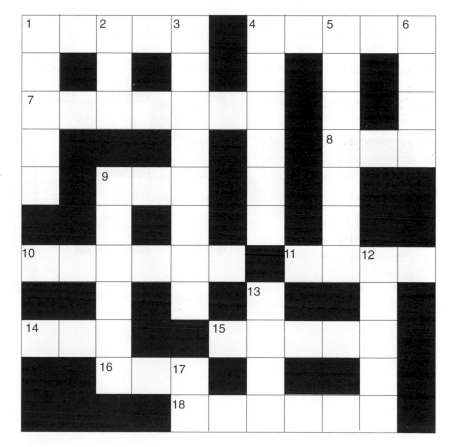

1 An expectant mother needs to eat **extra protein, vitamins and minerals**.

2 Nausea (feeling sick) during pregnancy can occur **at any time** of the day.

3 Heartburn is **a burning sensation in the chest** caused by acid in the stomach passing up into the gullet.

4 Hormones are substances which **help to regulate the way the body works**.

5 i   Pregnancy sickness – **usually disappears after the first three months**
  ii   Heartburn – **eat small meals and sleep propped up**
  iii   Constipation – **eat plenty of fruit, vegetables and fibre**
  iv   Varicose veins – **avoid standing for too long**

¹T	W	²I	N	³S		⁴B	I	⁵R	T	⁶H
U		U		H		R		U		E
⁷M	I	D	W	I	F	E		B		A
M				N		E		⁸E	D	D
Y		⁹E	G	G		C		L		
		M		L		H		L		
¹⁰B	A	B	I	E	S		¹¹C	A	¹²T	S
		R		S		¹³S			E	
¹⁴R	A	Y		¹⁵T	I	T	I	S		
		¹⁶O	V	¹⁷A		Z			T	
		¹⁸U	T	E	R	U	S			

(21 marks)

Total number of marks   29
First time score   ....
Score after revision   ....

1 About how much weight is gained, on average, during pregnancy?
A 6 kg
B 12 kg
C 18 kg
D 21 kg

2 Besides the enlarged uterus, name four other parts that help to increase the mother's weight during pregnancy:

i ....

ii ....

iii ....

iv ....

---

3 Label parts i–vi of the ultrasound scan of a baby at 12 weeks using the labels listed below:
amniotic fluid   placenta   uterus   body   head   leg

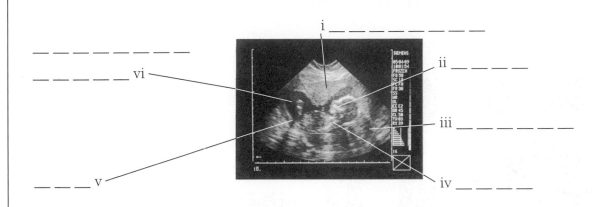

---

4 Tests given to the mother at the antenatal clinic include:
A eyesight test
B intelligence test
C saliva test
D urine test

5 At the first visit to the clinic the mother's blood is tested for
A anaemia, blood group, folic acid
B protein, blood group, Rhesus factor
C anaemia, blood group, Rhesus factor
D glucose, protein, blood group

6 Blood pressure is checked at every visit for a warning sign of
A hepatitis B
B anaemia
C infection
D pre-eclampsia

7 Pre-eclampsia
A occurs early in pregnancy
B only occurs in pregnancy
C never occurs during pregnancy
D always occurs in pregnancy

---

8 Match each test with the purpose of the investigation:

Test	Examines
i Nuchal translucency scan	three substances in the mother's blood
ii Chorionic villus sampling	fluid at the back of the baby's neck
iii Cordocentisis	cells from the placenta
iv Triple test	blood from the umbilical cord

1 About **12 kg** is gained, on average, during pregnancy.

2 The mother's weight is increased by the:
baby/foetus
placenta
umbilical cord
amniotic fluid/water

3 i **placenta**
   ii **head**
   iii **uterus**
   iv **body**
   v **leg**
   vi **amniotic fluid**

4 **Urine tests** are routine at the antenatal clinic. Glucose in the urine may indicate diabetes. If protein is present it may be an early sign of pre-eclampsia.

5 At the first visit to the clinic the mother's blood is tested for **anaemia, blood group, Rhesus factor**.

6 Blood pressure is checked for a warning sign of **pre-eclampsia** (toxaemia of pregnancy).

7 Pre-eclampsia **only occurs in pregnancy**.

8 i A **nuchal translucency scan** measures the **fluid at the back of the baby's neck**.
   ii **Chorionic villus sampling** investigates **cells from the placenta**.
   iii **Cordocentesis** removes a small sample of **blood from the umbilical cord**.
   iv The **triple test** investigates **three substances from the mother's blood**.

Total number of marks	19
First time score	....
Score after revision	....

1 Use the statements below to complete the lists of advantages of a hospital or home delivery.

familiar surroundings
more privacy than in a hospital ward
no domestic chores
nurses to help with the baby
not having to keep to a hospital routine

familiar doctor and midwife
restrictions on visitors
specialist equipment available
the family can be more involved
trained staff always present

Advantages of a hospital delivery

i   ....

ii   ....

iii   ....

iv   ....

v   ....

Advantages of a home delivery

i   ....

ii   ....

iii   ....

iv   ....

v   ....

2 Gynaecologists specialise in
 A the care of children's feet
 B the care of young children
 C pregnancy and childbirth
 D the female reproductive system

3 Obstetricians specialise in
 A the care of children's feet
 B the care of young children
 C pregnancy and childbirth
 D the female reproductive system

4 Paediatricians specialise in
 A the care of children's feet
 B the care of young children
 C pregnancy and childbirth
 D the female reproductive system

5 The birth plan is a plan:
 A of the hospital's maternity ward
 B prepared for a home birth
 C detailing the process of birth
 D prepared in accordance with the mother's preferences

Birthweight of live babies in grams (g)
☐ under 1500
▦ 1500–1999
▤ 2000–2499
▨ 2500–2999
▧ 3000–3499
▨ 3500 and over

39.5%   1.3%   1.6%   4.9%   17.1%   35.6%

6 From the pie chart above:

 i   the most common birthweight category is.. grams

 ii   the least common birthweight category is .... grams

7 Use a calculator to convert the birthweights from pounds (lb) to kilogrms (kg) for a baby weighing:

 i   4 lb = ... kg

 ii   6 lb = ... kg

 iii 8 lb = ... kg

 (Note: 2.2 lb = 1 kg; give answers to one decimal place.)

1 Five advantages of a hospital delivery:
no domestic chores
nurses to help with the baby
restrictions on visitors
specialist equipment available
trained staff always present

Five advantages of a home delivery:
familiar surroundings
more privacy than in a hospital ward
not having to keep to a hospital routine
familiar doctor and midwife
the family can be more involved

2 Gynaecologists specialise in **the female reproductive system**.

3 Obstetricians specialise in **pregnancy and childbirth**.

4 Paediatricians specialise in **the care of young children**.

5 The birth plan is **a plan prepared in accordance with the mother's preferences**.

6 i The most common birthweight category is **3500 grams and over**.
ii The least common birthweight category is **under 1500** grams.

7 A birthweight of:
i   4 lb = **1.8** kg
ii 6 lb = **2.7** kg
iii 8 lb = **3.6** kg

Total number of marks	19
Total number of marks	19
First time score	....
Score after revision	....

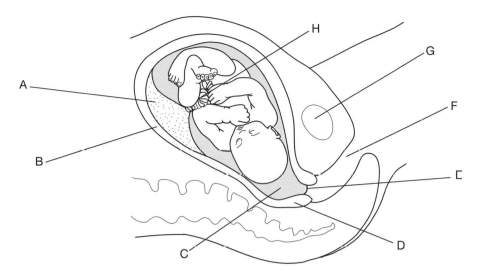

1   Is the first, second or third stage of labour shown in the diagram above? ....

2   Which of the parts A–G

   i   is liquid ('the waters')? ....

   ii   breaks to release 'the waters'? ....

   iii will become the afterbirth? ....

   iv   causes the contractions? ....

   v   will form the birth canal? (three answers) ...., ... and ....

   vi   is the pelvic bone? ....

   vii is the umbilical cord? ....

3   Give the technical name for 'the waters' ....

4   The baby's head emerging from the vagina is called ....

5   Name a way of relieving pain during labour which

   i   is taught in antenatal classes ....

   ii   is inhaled through a mouthpiece ....

   iii is injected into the lower part of the spine ....

   iv   requires electrodes to be placed on the skin ....

6   What is it called when

   i   the baby is born bottom first (two words)?...

   ii   an instrument like large tongs is used (two words)?..

   iii the baby is removed through the abdominal wall (two words)?.......................................

   iv   the process of labour is started artificially (one word)?..

1 The diagram shows **the first stage of labour**.

2 i　Part **C** (**amniotic fluid**) is liquid.
　　ii　Part **E** (**amnion**) breaks to release 'the waters'.
　　iii　Part **A** (**placenta**) will become the afterbirth.
　　iv　Part **B** (**uterus**) causes the contractions.
　　v　Parts **B** (**uterus**), **D** (**cervix**) and **F** (**vagina**) form the birth canal.
　　vi　Part **G** is the pelvic bone.　　　　　　　　　　　　(9 marks)
　　vii　Part **H** is the umbilical cord.

3 **Amniotic fluid** is the technical name for 'the waters'.

4 When the baby's head emerges from the vagina it is called **crowning**.

5 i　**Relaxation/breathing exercises** are taught in antenatal classes.
　　ii　**Gas-and-air** is inhaled through a mouthpiece.
　　iii　**Epidural anaesthetic** is injected into the lower part of the spine.
　　iv　**TENS** requires electrodes to be placed on the skin.

6 i　The baby is born bottom first in a **breech birth**.　　　(2 marks)
　　ii　An instrument like large tongs is used in a **forceps delivery**.　(2 marks)
　　iii　The baby is removed through the abdominal wall in a **caesarian section**.　(2 marks)
　　iv　**Induction** is the process of starting labour artificially.　(1 marks)

Total number of marks　23
First time score　.......
Score after revision　.......

1 Match the five checks carried out on a baby immediately after birth with the healthy response:

Check	Healthy response
i pulse	pink colour
ii activity	breathing well
iii respiration	vigorous crying
iv appearance	over 100 beats per minute
v response to stimuli (e.g. touch)	active movements

2 In the routine examination of newborn babies, why

i   are the fingers and toes counted? ....

....

ii   is the mouth checked? ....

....

iii   are the hip joints examined? ....

....

3 After the baby is born, the birth must be registered with the
A Hospital
B Family court
C Social Security department
D Registrar of births, marriages and deaths

4 Babies have to be registered by the parents within
A 2 weeks of birth
B 4 weeks of birth
C 6 weeks of birth
D 8 weeks of birth

5 The baby receives a medical card
A from the local Health Authority
B from a postnatal clinic
C when a birth certificate is issued
D from the hospital, doctor or midwife who delivered the baby

6 A few days after birth, a few drops of blood are taken from a baby's heel to test for
A PKU and thyroxine
B thyroxine and blood group
C blood group and red cell count
D red cell count and PKU

7 Babies who lack thyroxine will:
A grow normally but have learning difficulties
B need physiotherapy
C be undersized and have learning difficulties
D need a special diet

8 Babies with PKU will:
A grow normally but have learning difficulties
B need physiotherapy
C be undersized and have learning difficulties
D need a special diet

1   i   pulse – **over 100 beats per minute**
       ii   activity – **active movements**
       iii   respiration – **breathing well**
       iv   appearance – **pink colour**
       v   response to stimuli (e.g. touch) – **vigorous crying**

2   i   Fingers and toes are counted because occasionally there is **an extra one**.
       ii   The mouth is checked for **cleft palate**.
       iii   The hip joints are examined to check for **dislocation of the hip**.

3   After the baby is born, the birth must be registered with the **Registrar of births, marriages and deaths**.

4   Babies have to be registered by the parents within **6 weeks of birth**.

5   The baby receives a medical card **when a birth certificate is issued**.

6   A few days after birth, a few drops of blood are taken from a baby's heel to test for **PKU and thyroxine**.

7   Babies who lack thyroxine will **be undersized and have learning difficulties** unless given thyroxine from an early age.

8   Babies with PKU **will need a special diet**.

Total number of marks   14
First time score   ....
Score after revision   ....

SECTION 3 CARING FOR BABIES

CONTENTS

1 Fill in the missing words:

The newborn baby shows the stump of the

u _ _ _ _ _ _ _ _ _   c _ _ _. This will

fall off in a few days leaving the n _ _ _ _. The

arrow points to the f _ _ _ _ _ _ _ _ _ _ _ (soft spot) where the b _ _ _ _ of the skull

have not yet joined together. The soft spot is covered by a very tough membrane which protects the

b _ _ _ _ underneath.

At birth, the baby's body may be covered with a greasy, whitish substance called

v _ _ _ _ _. New babies may also develop whitish-yellow spots on the face called

m _ _ _ _ (milk spots). These are caused by blocked oil g _ _ _ _ _ in the skin. In

many newborn babies, the skin and eyes become tinged with yellow for a few days. This condition

is called j _ _ _ _ _ _ _. 'Stork bites' (red blotches) on the skin of some babies are another

name for b _ _ _ _ m _ _ _ _.

2 Full-term babies are those born at:
   A about 40 weeks
   B any time after 30 weeks
   C any time after 36 weeks
   D 42 weeks or more

3 Perinatal is the term used for the:
   A 28th week of pregnancy to 1 month after birth
   B the day before the birth to the day after
   C 39th week of pregnancy to 1 week after birth
   D whole of pregnancy to 1 week after birth

4 The terms below describe children in different age groups. Use these numbers to fill in the blank spaces.

1   1   1   2½   2½   4   4   5   6   6

neonate –   birth to .... weeks

infant –   from......... weeks to......... year

young baby –   the first .... months

older baby –   from .... months to .... year

toddler –   from .... year to .... years

pre-school –   from .... years to .... years

5 Tick those conditions in the mother that may prevent the unborn baby from growing properly
   ☐ smoking
   ☐ having a high alcohol intake
   ☐ taking drugs
   ☐ not eating enough

6 Which measurement is not taken shortly after birth?
   A head circumference
   B height
   C length
   D weight

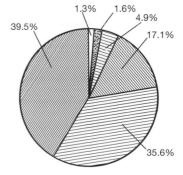

Birthweight in grams
☐ under 1500
▦ 1500–1999
▤ 2000–2499
▨ 2500–2999
▧ 3000–3499
▨ 3500 and over

39.5%   1.3%   1.6%   4.9%   17.1%   35.6%

7 Using the pie chart, give the percentage of babies whose full-term birthweight is:

   i   3500 g or over ....

   ii   less than 2000 g ....

1 The drawing of the newborn baby shows the stump of the **umbilical cord**. This will fall off in a few days leaving the **navel**. The arrow points to the **fontanelle** (soft spot) where the **bones** of the skull have not yet joined together. The soft spot is covered by a very tough membrane which protects the **brain** underneath.

At birth, the baby's body may be covered with a greasy, whitish substance called **vernix**. New babies may also develop whitish-yellow spots on the face called **milia** (milk spots). These are caused by blocked oil **glands** in the skin. In many newborn babies, the skin and eyes become tinged with yellow for a few days. This condition is called **jaundice**. 'Stork bites' (red blotches) on the skin of some babies are another name for **birth marks**.

(10 marks)

2 Full-term babies are those born at **about 40 weeks**.

3 Perinatal is the term used for the time from about the **28th week of pregnancy to 1 month after birth**.

4 neonate – birth to **4 weeks**
infant – from **4** weeks to **1** year
young baby – the first **6** months
older baby – from **6** months to **1** year
toddler – from **1** year to **2½** years
pre-school – from **2½** years to **5** years. (10 marks)

5 When the mother **smokes, has a high alcohol intake, takes drugs** or **does not eat enough**, her unborn baby may be prevented from growing properly. (4 marks)

6 **Height** is not measured until a child is old enough to stand upright.

7 i **39.5%** of babies have a birthweight of 3500 g (35 kg) or above.
ii **2.9%** of babies have a birthweight of less than 2000 g (1.3% + 1.6% = 2.9%).

Total number of marks	29
First time score	....
Score after revision	....

1 Is a normal newborn baby

	Yes	No
i aware of sounds		
ii unable to swallow		
iii aware of unpleasant smells		
iv aware of pain		
v able to suck the thumb		
vi unable to see		
vii short-sighted		
viii long-sighted		
ix sensitive to taste		
x able to yawn?		

2 Primitive reflexes shown by a new baby (e.g., grasping and walking movements)
A are acquired after birth
B are inborn and automatic
C need to be taught
D gradually become automatic

3 By about what age have the primitive reflexes usually disappeared?
A 3 months
B 4 months
C 5 months
D 6 months

4 Cot death is the term often used for:
A any death in a cot
B death caused by an unsafe cot
C expected death of an infant
D sudden, unexpected infant death with no obvious cause

5 Cot death is the term often used for:
A IDSS
B DISS
C SIDS
D ISDS

6 The risk of cot death is reduced when the baby
A is exposed to tobacco smoke
B does not become over-hot
C is placed on the front to sleep
D is bottle-fed

7 The recommended temperature for the room in which a baby sleeps is:
A 16–20°C
B 20–24°C
C 14–18°C
D 18–22°C

8 It is recommended that babies sleep:
A face downwards
B on their backs
C on their right side
D on their left side

9 As the graph below shows, the number of cot deaths has been falling since ...., with the fall being greatest between .... and ....

10 Calculate the reduction in cot deaths between:
   i   1989 and 2002 ....
   ii   1991 and 1992 ....
   iii 2001 and 2002 ....

Sudden infant deaths in babies under the age of 1 year in England & Wales.

(*Source: Foundation for the Study of Infant Deaths*)

Graph data: 1989: 1367, 1990: 1234, 1991: 1047, 1992: 559, 1993: 473, 1994: 476, 1995: 416, 1996: 468, 1997: 393, 1998: 286, 1999: 280, 2000: 246, 2001: 247, 2002: 192

1 A normal newborn baby is:

i	aware of sounds	Yes
ii	unable to swallow	No
iii	aware of unpleasant smells	Yes
iv	aware of pain	Yes
v	able to suck the thumb	Yes
vi	unable to see	No
vii	short-sighted	Yes
viii	long-sighted	No
ix	sensitive to taste	Yes
x	able to yawn	Yes

(10 marks)

2 The primitive reflexes shown by a baby **are inborn and automatic**.

3 Primitive reflexes have usually disappeared by **3 months**.

4 Cot death is the term often used to describe **sudden, unexpected infant death with no obvious cause**.

5 Cot death is the term often used for **SIDS** (Sudden Infant Death Syndrome).

6 The risk of cot death is reduced when the baby **does not become over-hot**.

7 The recommended temperature for the room in which a baby sleeps is **16–20°C**.

8 The recommended position for babies to sleep is **on their backs**.

9 The number of cot deaths has been falling since **1989**, with the fall being greatest between **1991** and **1992**.

(2 marks)

10 The reduction in cot deaths between:
  i   1989 and 2002 was **1175**
  ii 1991 and 1992 was **488**.
  iii 2001 and 2002 was **55**.

Total number of marks   22
First time score   ....
Score after revision   ....

All babies need:			
love	warmth	fresh air	protection
food	shelter	sunlight	medical care
rest	clothing	cleanliness	companionship
play	exercise		

1 From the words in the box:

 i   name one which helps a baby to develop emotionally: ....

 ii name one which helps a baby to develop socially: ....

 iii name one which helps a baby to develop intellectually: ....

 iv name six that are essential for the baby to survive and to grow and develop physically:

   ....

   ....

   ....

2 Complete this wordsearch by finding the 14 needs of a baby in the box above. The words can be horizontal, vertical, diagonal or back to front.

V	A	R	Z	I	S	U	N	L	I	G	H	T	E	T	A
M	E	D	I	C	A	L	C	A	R	E	O	G	Z	E	W
E	Y	B	S	K	C	C	Q	D	C	Y	Y	M	I	D	A
L	A	E	V	O	L	O	W	B	S	L	A	O	X	U	R
T	C	X	I	E	E	F	A	S	R	F	G	C	I	U	M
D	C	O	M	P	A	N	I	O	N	S	H	I	P	A	T
C	D	G	U	Z	N	Y	M	W	P	V	U	Z	T	D	H
L	X	S	P	A	L	S	B	R	Q	V	O	R	Q	P	Y
O	S	A	Y	O	I	N	O	J	S	H	E	L	T	E	R
T	M	Z	L	U	N	T	K	U	J	E	V	I	X	C	H
H	I	W	S	F	E	C	F	R	E	S	H	A	I	R	G
I	H	T	A	C	S	F	O	Q	E	D	H	O	E	K	P
N	J	E	T	C	S	A	O	E	D	W	F	S	B	M	C
G	A	I	N	L	R	J	D	G	Z	T	T	N	I	Y	X
W	O	B	R	F	V	D	U	E	S	I	C	R	E	X	E
N	A	H	P	L	A	Y	N	T	P	A	Z	B	S	R	D

1 i **Love** helps the emotional development of a baby.

ii **Companionship** helps a baby to develop socially.

iii The stimulation from **play** helps the intellectual development of a baby.

iv The following are essential for the baby to survive and to grow and develop physically:

food	clothing	cleanliness
rest	exercise	protection
warmth	fresh air	medical care
shelter	sunlight	

(Six answers only are required) (6 marks)

2

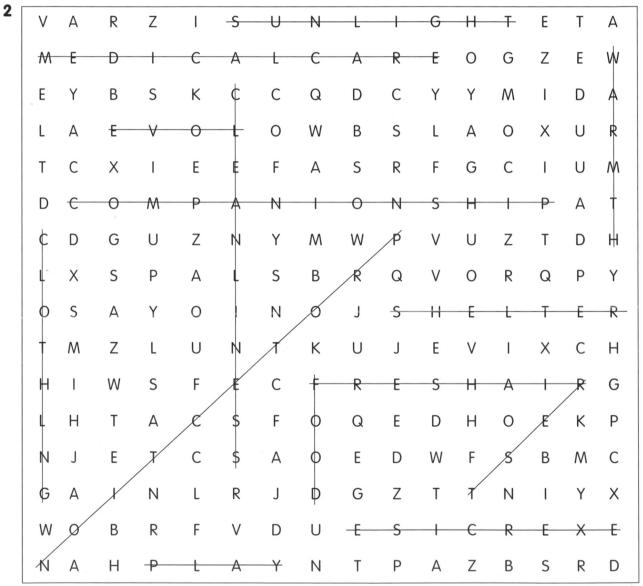

(14 marks)

Total number of marks	23
First time score	....
Score after revision	....

1 To stop a baby from crying should you
   A shout at the baby
   B shake the baby
   C smack the baby
   D do none of the above?

2 Letting young babies cry for a long time without attending to them will:
   A not affect them
   B teach them to be patient
   C cause them distress
   D prevent them from becoming spoilt

3 Babies are able to shed tears when they cry
   A from birth
   B by 1 week old
   C by 3–4 weeks old
   D by 3–4 months old

4 A young baby may cry because it is hungry every
   A 1–2 hours
   B 2–3 hours
   C 3–4 hours
   D 2–5 hours

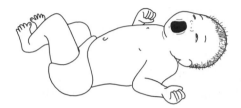

5 Baby Ben wouldn't stop crying. His mother knew he wasn't hungry, but:

  i   was he thirsty? Are breast- or bottle-fed babies likely to get more thirsty? ....

  ii was he in pain? Give two ways in which babies cry when in pain:

     (a) .... (b) ....

  iii does he dislike the dark? What sort of light could be left on?..

  iv does he feel lonely? How can his mother find out?...

  v   is he uncomfortable? Suggest three things she might check:

     (a)...

     (b)...

     (c)...

  vi is he tired? What movements could encourage him to sleep?..

  vii what types of audio tape might encourage him to sleep? Give two suggestions:

     (a) .... (b) ....

6 Colic is a common cause of crying in young babies. Colic is .... in the abdomen.

7 i   At what time of day does crying due to colic mainly occur? ....

    ii By what age has the crying due to colic usually ceased? ....

1 **None of the above**. Shouting at, shaking or smacking a baby will frighten or hurt the baby, but not stop the crying.

2 Letting young babies cry for a long time without attending to them will **cause them distress**. At this stage they are too young to learn.

3 Tears are not usually shed until a baby is **3–4 weeks old**.

4 A young baby may cry because it is hungry at any time from about **2–5 hours** after the last feed.

5 i **Bottle-fed** babies are likely to get more thirsty than breast-fed babies.
 ii When in pain babies may
  (a) **cry loudly** (b) **whimper**.
 iii **A dim light** can be left on for babies who dislike the dark.
 iv A baby who feels lonely will be comforted by being **picked up / cuddled / spoken to**.
 v Babies can cry with discomfort for a number of reasons:
  a wet or soiled nappy / being too hot / being too cold / a bright light shining in the eyes / wind / teething. (3 marks)
 vi **Rocking / massage** may soothe a baby and encourage sleep.
 vii Audio tapes of **soft music / repetitive sounds / sounds similar to those the baby heard in the womb** may encourage sleep. (2 marks)

6 Colic is **pain** in the abdomen.

7 i Crying due to colic mainly occurs **in the evening**.
 ii The crying has usually ceased by the age of **3 months**.

Total number of marks	18
Total number of marks	18
First time score	....
Score after revision	....

1 The natural food for babies is:
A cows' milk
B breast milk
C formula milk
D infant milk

2 Which contains the right amounts of all the food substances for a young baby?
A cows' milk
B breast milk
C formula milk
D infant milk

3 Which is easiest for a baby to digest?
A cows' milk
C breast milk
C formula milk
D infant milk

4 Which contains antibodies to help protect a baby against disease?
A cows' milk
B breast milk
C formula milk
D infant milk

5 Comparison of breast milk and cows' milk (grams per 100 ml)

	Sugar	Fat	Protein	Minerals (including salt)	Water
Breast milk	7	4	1.2	0.4	90
Cows' milk	4.7	4	3.3	0.75	88

i   Which milk contains the most water?............
ii Which milk is sweeter? ....
iii Which has a higher mineral content? ....
iv Which has a higher protein content? ....

6 Cows' milk is less easy for young babies to digest because:
A cows' milk contains much less water
B cows' milk has a higher fat content
C the fat droplets are smaller
D the type of protein differs from that in breast milk

7 Cows' milk is 'too strong' for young babies because it contains too much:
A fat
B sugar
C protein
D salt

8 A danger of giving babies too much salt is:
A it will make them too thirsty
B it gives them indigestion
C they will not take the milk
D their kidneys may be unable to remove the excess

9 If, in an emergency, a baby has to be given cows' milk, is it safer to
A dilute with water
B dilute with water and add a little sugar
C dilute with water and add salt
D add sugar and salt?

10 The type of sugar found in milk is:
A glucose
B sucrose
C lactose
D fructose

11 Gastro-enteritis is:
A indigestion and sickness
B sickness and diarrhoea
C diarrhoea and indigestion
D sickness and vomiting

12 Gastro-enteritis rarely occurs in babies:
A who are breast-fed
B fed on infant formula
C who are bottle-fed
D given extra vitamins

13 A little cows' milk can be given at:
A 3 months old
B 6 months old
C 9 months old
D 1 year old

14 Cows' milk can replace breast/formula milk at:
A 3 months old
B 6 months old
C 9 months old
D 1 year old

1 **Breast milk** is the natural food for babies.

2 **Breast milk** contains the right amounts of all the necessary food substances for a young baby.

3 **Breast milk** is easiest for a baby to digest.

4 **Breast milk** contains antibodies to help protect a baby against disease.

5 i   **Breast milk** contains more water than cows' milk.
    ii   **Breast milk** is sweeter.
    iii **Cows' milk** has a higher mineral content.
    iv **Cows' milk** has a higher protein content.

6 Cows' milk is less easy for young babies to digest because **the type of protein differs from that in breast milk**.

7 Cow's milk is 'too strong' for young babies because it contains too much **salt**.

8 A danger of giving young babies too much salt is that **their kidneys may be unable to remove the excess**.

9 If, in an emergency, a baby has to be given cows' milk, is it safer to **dilute it with water and add a little sugar**. Breast milk is sweeter than cows' milk.

10 The type of sugar found in milk is **lactose**.

11 Gastro-enteritis is **sickness and diarrhoea**.

12 Gastro-enteritis rarely occurs in young babies **who are breast-fed**.

13 Babies can be given a little cows' milk when **6 months old**, for example on breakfast cereals or in sauces and custards.

14 Cows' milk can replace breast milk or formula milk at **1 year old**.

Total number of marks	17
First time score	....
Score after revision	....

1 Add these words to labels i–vii to the diagram of the breast :

areola

fatty tissue

milk gland

nipple

opening of milk duct

reservoir for storing milk

skin

i _ _ _ _ _

ii _ _ _ _ _ _ _ _ _ _ _

iii _ _ _ _ _ _ _ _ _ _ _

iv _

_ _ _ _

v _ _ _ _ _ _

vi _

vii _ _ _ _ _ _ _

2 The size of the breasts before pregnancy is an indication of
  A the amount of fatty tissue present
  B the number of milk-producing glands
  C the size of the milk storage reservoirs
  D whether the mother will be able to breast-feed

3 Before producing milk, breasts produce:
  A lactose
  B sucrose
  C colostrum
  D casein

4 After giving birth, how long is it before milk is produced?
  A 1–2 days
  B 2–3 days
  C 3–4 days
  D 4–5 days

5 Is it usual to feed a young baby
  A whenever the baby cries and seems hungry
  B by keeping to a strict routine
  C at times which suit the mother
  D as directed by the health visitor?

6 How many times may a three-day-old baby want to be fed in 24 hours?
  A 4–6
  B 6–8
  C 8–10
  D 10–12

7 When they settle down, most newborn babies want to be fed
  A twice a day
  B about 4 times a day
  C about 6 times a day
  D about 8 times a day

8 It is recommended that mothers exclusively breast-feed for
  A 12 months
  B 9 months
  C 6 months
  D 2 months

9 It is recommended that weaning starts at about
  A 3 months
  B 4 months
  C 6 months
  D 9 months

10 Tick the advantages of breast-feeding:

the baby is less likely to become overweight

the baby is less likely to become constipated

the baby is less likely to develop nappy rash

it is cheaper than infant formula

it gives time for a bond of attachment to develop

the mother's uterus shrinks back to size more quickly

the baby is less likely to develop allergies

1   i   **skin**
        ii   **milk gland**
        iii **fatty tissue**
        iv   **reservoir for storing milk**
        v   **nipple**
        vi   **opening of milk duct**
        vii **areola**

2   The size of the breasts before pregnancy is an indication of **the amount of fatty tissue present**.

3   Before producing milk, breasts produce **colostrum**.

4   Milk is produced **2–3 days** after giving birth.

5   It is usual to feed a baby **whenever the baby cries and seems hungry**.

6   Between the 3rd and 6th days after birth, a baby may want to be fed **10–12** times in 24 hours. The more the baby sucks, the more the breasts are stimulated to produce a good supply of milk.

7   When they settle down, most newborn babies want to be fed **about 6 times a day**.

8   It is recommended that mothers exclusively breast-feed for **6 months**, i.e. that breast milk is the only source of food for the the first 6 months.

9   It is recommended that weaning starts at about **6 months**.

10   Advantages of breast-feeding:

the baby is less likely to become overweight	✓
the baby is less likely to be constipated	✓
the baby is less likely to develop nappy rash	✓
it is cheaper than infant formula	✓
it gives time for a bond of attachment to develop	✓
the mother's uterus shrinks back to size more quickly	✓
the baby is less likely to develop allergies, e.g. eczema and asthma	✓

Total number of marks	22
First time score	....
Score after revision	....

1 Tick the four essential rules for bottle-feeding from the list below:

use the right type of milk

give the baby a variety of different milks

cuddle the baby while it is being fed

leave the baby to feed itself

follow instructions for making up the feed

use more milk powder for a hungry baby

keep all equipment scrupulously clean

sterilise the equipment once a week

2 Feeding bottles need:

i   a wide neck for easy ....

ii to be made of clear ....

iii a cap to keep the .... clean

iv graduated measurements in ....

    and ....

3 The way the milk powder is being measured in the diagram is:

A the wrong way
B the right way
C unnecessary
D the right way if the powder has been pressed down hard

4 Babies can get gastro-enteritis when:

A boiled water is used to mix the feed
B the equipment used is sterilised properly
C the feed is stored in a warm place
D the teat is protected from contamination

5 Give three reasons why a baby should not be left to feed itself:

i...

....

ii..

....

iii...

....

6 When mixing a feed it is important to:

A mix the water and milk powder together before putting it in the bottle
B put the powder in the bottle before the water
C put the water in the bottle before the powder
D mix the powder with boiling water

7 The hole in the teat should allow the milk to

A drip out slowly
B drip out rapidly
C flow out
D flow out only when the bottle is pressed

8 One way to check that the milk is not too hot for the baby to drink is to sprinkle a few drops on the:

A back of the hand
B palm of the hand
C inside of the wrist
D forearm

9 Sometimes a baby needs to be helped to bring up wind. 'Wind'

A is an air bubble from the baby's stomach
B an air bubble from the baby's lungs
C only occurs with breast-fed babies
D only occurs with bottle-fed babies

1 Four essential rules for bottle-feeding:
use the right type of milk
cuddle the baby while it is being fed
follow instructions for making up the feed
keep all equipment scrupulously clean.

2 Feeding bottles need:
i a wide neck for easy **cleaning**
ii to be made of clear **material / glass / plastic**
iii a cap to keep the **teat** clean
iv graduated measurements in **millilitres** (ml) and **fluid ounces** (fl oz).

3 The way the milk powder is being measured in the diagram is **the right way.**

4 Babies can get gastro-enteritis when the **feed is stored in a warm place.**

5 Reasons why a baby should not be left to feed itself are (three answers only required):
the baby might choke
to prevent the baby sucking on an flattened teat
to prevent the baby sucking on an empty bottle
the baby is deprived of the comfort of being held close
there will be no-one to help the baby bring up wind. (3 marks)

6 When mixing a feed it is important to **put the water in the bottle before the powder** to obtain the exact quantities of water and powder.

7 The hole in the teat should allow the milk to **drip out rapidly.**

8 To check that the milk is not too hot for the baby to drink, sprinkle a few drops on to the **inside of the wrist.**

9 'Wind' **is an air bubble from the baby's stomach.**

Total number of marks	18
First time score	....
Score after revision	....

NUTRITIONAL INFORMATION typical values per 100 ml prepared feed		
	First milk	**Follow-on milk**
Energy	285 kj/68 kcal	285 kj/68 kcal
Protein	1.45 g	2.1 g
Sugar	6.9 g	7.4 g
Fat	3.82 g	3.4 g
Minerals		
Calcium	39 mg	72 mg
Chloride	40 mg	58 mg
Iron	0.6 mg	1.2 mg
Sodium	17 mg	30 mg
Vitamins		
Vitamin A	82.0 µg	80.0 µg
B vitamins	137 µg	245 µg
Vitamin C	6.9 mg	10 mg
Vitamin D	1.0 µg	1.1 µg
Vitamin E	0.4 mg	0.5 mg
Vitamin K	2.7 µg	2.9 µg

1 Comparing first milk with follow-on milk, which:

i   is for younger babies? ....

ii   is for older babies? ....

iii   contains more fat? ....

iv   is sweeter? ....

2 Which occurs in the largest amounts?
A   vitamin A   C   vitamin D
B   vitamin C   D   vitamin K

3 Which elements indicate the presence of salt?
A   calcium and chloride
B   chloride and iron
C   iron and sodium
D   sodium and chloride

4 Which dietary item is absent in milk?
A   protein   C   fat
B   carbohydrate   D   fibre

TYPICAL FEEDING GUIDE						
Approximate age	Approximate weight		Number of feeds per 24 hours	Level scoops of powder per feed (1 scoop = 5 g)	Quantity of water per feed	
	kg	lb			ml	fluid oz
0–1 week	3	7	6	3	80	3
2–4 weeks	3.5		6	4	110	4
1–2 months	4.5		5	5	140	5
3 months	5.5		5	6	170	6
4–5 months	6.5		5	6	170	6
6 months	8		4	7	200	7
7–12 months	8.5+		3	7	200	7

5 In the feeding guide, complete the column for the weight of babies in pounds (lb) when 1 kg = 2.2 lb, giving your answers to the nearest pound.

6 Using the feeding guide above, give the:

i   average weight of a baby aged 6 months: ....kg

ii   number of feeds per day at 3 months: ....

iii   amount of water for 3 scoops of formula: ....ml

iv   the amount of formula for 200 ml water: ....g

7 The number of milk feeds begins to be reduced at 6 months because:
A   the baby needs less food
B   the baby is growing less quickly
C   weaning has started
D   more milk is taken per feed

8 Salt is not added to milk because:
A   babies do not need salt
B   babies do not like salt
C   milk already contains enough salt
D   the milk tastes better without salt

1 Comparing 100 ml of first milk with the same quantity of follow-on milk:
   i   **first milk** is recommended for babies under 6 months of age
   ii   **follow-on milk** is recommended for babies older than 6 months
   iii **first milk** contains a little more fat
   iv **follow-on milk** is a little sweeter.

2 The vitamin present in the largest amounts in formula milk is **vitamin C**.
Note: 1000 micrograms (μg) = 1 milligram (mg).

3 **Sodium and chloride** indicate the presence of salt (sodium chloride).

4 **Fibre** is absent in milk. It is present in fruit, vegetables and cereals, and becomes part of a baby's diet when weaning begins. Note: carbohydrate is present in milk in the form of sugar.

5

kg	lb
3.5	**8**
4.5	**10**
5.5	**12**
6.5	**14**
8	**18**
8.5+	**19+**

6 i   The average weight of a baby at 6 months is **8** kg.
   ii   The number of feeds per day at 3 months is **5**.
   iii The amount of water for 3 scoops of formula is **80** ml.
   iv The amount of formula in grams for 200 ml water is **35** g (7 scoops at 5 g per scoop).

7 The number of milk feeds begins to be reduced at 6 months because **weaning has started** and the baby is taking in other foods besides milk.

8 Salt is not added to milk because **milk already contains enough salt**.

Total number of marks	19
First time score	....
Score after revision	....

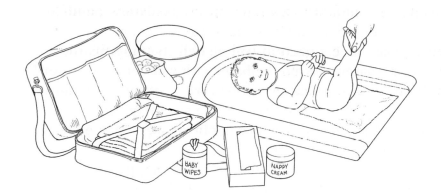

1   Use lines to match the two parts of each sentence:

    Changing a nappy

    i   Place the baby on a flat surface
    ii   Using a changing mat
    iii After removing a wet nappy
    iv   After removing a dirty nappy
    v   Put used terry nappies
    vi   Wrap up disposable nappies

    in a bucket containing sterilising solution
    clean the baby's skin with cotton wool and warm water
    before placing in a nappy sack or bin
    wipe the baby with wet cotton wool or baby wipes helps prevent soiling objects underneath
    to allow both of the carer's hands to be free for nappy changing

2   The main purpose of nappy cream is to:
    A   clean the baby's bottom
    B   make the baby smell nice
    C   keep the baby's bottom soft
    D   help to prevent nappy rash

3   Which of the following is not recommended for use when washing nappies and baby clothes?
    A   soap
    B   boiling
    C   sterilising solution
    D   biological detergents

4   Cleanliness is very important up to the age of:
    A   3 months
    B   6 months
    C   9 months
    D   1 year

5   There is evidence that an older baby's immunity can be reduced by:
    A   getting dirty when playing
    B   mixing with other children
    C   visiting the baby clinic
    D   keeping the baby too clean

6   Place these signs of nappy rash in the order of their appearance: septic spots, red skin, red rash, rough skin

    i   ....
    ii   ....
    iii ....
    iv   ....

7   Nappy rash is caused by:
    A   ammonia   C   antibiotics
    B   allergy   D   antibodies

8   Breast-fed babies are less prone to nappy rash because their stools are:
    A   less acidic   C   harder
    B   more acidic   D   softer

9   Children should be able to start to wipe the nose by the age of:
    A   2 years   C   4 years
    B   3 years   D   5 years

1   i   Place the baby on a flat surface – **to allow both of the carer's hands to be free for nappy changing**.

    ii   Using a changing mat – **helps prevent soiling objects underneath.**

    iii   After removing a wet nappy – **wipe the baby with wet cotton wool or baby wipes.**

    iv   After removing a dirty nappy – **clean the skin with cotton wool and warm water.**

    v   Put used terry nappies – **in a bucket containing sterilising solution.**

    vi   Wrap up disposable nappies – **before placing in a nappy sack or bin.**

2   The main purpose of nappy cream is to **help to prevent nappy rash**.

3   **Biological detergents** are not recommended for use when washing nappies and baby clothes because they may irritate the baby's skin.

4   Cleanliness is very important up to the age of **6 months**. By this time the baby's immune system should be well developed.

5   There is evidence that an older baby's immunity can be reduced by **keeping the baby too clean**.

6   Signs of nappy rash in the order of their appearance are:

    i   **red skin**

    ii   **red rash**

    iii   **rough skin**

    iv   **septic spots**.

7   Nappy rash is caused by **ammonia** produced from urine when urine comes into contact with bacteria in the stools.

8   Breast-fed babies are less prone to nappy rash because their stools are **more acidic**.

9   Children should be able to start to wipe the nose by the age of **2 years**.

Total number of marks	17
First time score	....
Score after revision	....

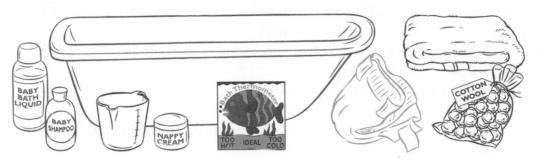

1 List the eight items around the bath in the order that they will be used during bathtime (do not include the bath).

i ....   v ....

ii ....   vi ....

iii ....   vii ....

iv..   viii ....

2 Why is this mother putting her elbow in the bath water but not the baby?

....

....

3 How is the baby being held securely in the bath?

....

....

4 The temperature of the room in which the baby is being bathed should be:
   A about 37°C
   B more than 37°C
   C about 20°C
   D less than 20°C

5 The bathwater should be:
   A about 37°C
   B more than 37°C
   C about 20°C
   D less than 20°C

6 Are the statements below correct practice when bathing a baby?

	YES	NO
i Use soap to wash the baby's face		
ii Clean the eyes everyday		
iii Use cotton buds to clean the ears		
iv Shampoo the hair every day		
v Wash the baby's bottom before its face		
vi Do not try to retract the foreskin of a baby boy		
vii Rub the baby dry		
viii Dry creases in the skin properly or they can become sore		

1 The order in which the item will be used during bathtime:
  i   undress the baby and wrap in a warm **towel**
  ii   use a **bath thermometer** to check the temperature of the bath water
  iii use **cotton wool** to wash the baby's face
  iv   use **baby shampoo** to wash the baby's hair
  v   use a **jug** for water to rinse the baby's hair
  iv   add **baby bath liquid** to the bath water before putting the baby in the bath
  vii apply **nappy cream** to the baby's bottom
  viii put on the **nappy**.

2 The elbow can be used **to test the temperature of the bath water** before placing the baby in the bath.

3 One of the mother's hands **holds the baby's shoulder**.

4 The temperature of the room in which the baby is being bathed should be **about 20°C**.

5 The bathwater should be **about 37°C**.

6 Correct practice when bathing a baby:
  i   **No**, soap is not used to wash the baby's face.
  ii   **No**, only clean the eyes if infected or sticky.
  iii **No**, cotton buds can easily damage the ear drums.
  iv   **No**, shampooing the hair once or twice a week is enough.
  v   **No**, the baby's face should be washed first to prevent the transfer of germs from the baby's bottom to the face.
  vi   **Yes**, the foreskin of a baby boy is not yet separate from the tip of the penis. Attempts to retract (draw back) the foreskin may cause bleeding.
  vii **No**, pat gently until dry, but do not rub.
  viii **Yes**, creases in the skin can become sore if not properly dried.

Total number of marks	20
First time score	....
Score after revision	....

1 Use lines to match these statements in pairs:

Baby clothes should:

i   be non-irritant

ii be flame-resistant

iii not cramp the feet

iv avoid open-weave garments

v   avoid drawstrings near the baby's neck

young toes easily become deformed

a strand caught round a finger could damage it

will not scratch or irritate the skin

if pulled too tight they can strangle

will not easily catch fire

2 Say whether each of these materials is natural (N) or synthetic (S)

acrylic ...., cotton ...., nylon ...., polyester ...., viscose ...., wool ....

3 Place each of the materials in question 2 in the most appropriate space below:

i   used for nappies ....

ii crease resistant ....

iii very strong ....

iv warm to wear ....

v   an alternative to wool ....

vi lacks strength ....

4 Use these labels to identify the fabric care symbols:

three dots – hot temperature

unsuitable for dry cleaning

maximum temperature of the water is 60°C

reduced machine action for synthetics

much reduced machine action for wool

do not iron

do not wash

do not bleach

handwash only

may be tumble-dried

i ....

ii ....

iii ....

iv ....

v ....

vi ....

vii ....

viii ....

ix ....

x ....

1 Baby clothes should:
   i   be non-irritant – **will not scratch or irritate the skin**
   ii be flame-resistant – **will not easily catch fire**
   iii not cramp the feet – **young toes easily become deformed**
   iv avoid drawstrings near the baby's neck – **if pulled too tight they can strangle**
   v avoid open-weave garments – **a strand of wool caught tight around a baby's finger could damage it** by cutting off the blood supply.

2 Natural materials – **cotton** and **wool**
Synthetic materials – **acrylic**, **nylon**, **polyester** and **viscose**.   (6 marks)

3 i   used for nappies – **cotton**   iv warm to wear – **wool**
    ii crease resistant – **polyester**   v   an alternative to wool – **acrylic**
    iii very strong – **nylon**   vi lacks strength – **viscose**   (6 marks)

4   Fabric care symbols:

    i   maximum temperature of the water is 60°C
    ii   reduced machine action for synthetics
    iii much reduced machine action for wool
    iv handwash only
    v   do not wash
    vi may be tumble-dried
    vii do not bleach
    viii three dots – hot temperature
    ix do not iron
    x   unsuitable for dry cleaning

Total number of marks   27
First time score   ....
Score after revision   ....

1 To prevent the baby's head from being caught between the bars of the cot, the bars should be:

A 45–65 mm apart

B 55–75 mm apart

C 65–75 mm apart

D 75–85 mm apart

2 To prevent the baby's arms and legs from being trapped in the gap around the mattress, the gap should be no more than:

A 40 mm

B 50 mm

C 60 mm

D 70 mm

3 Duvets are not recommended for babies because:

A they are too warm

B they are not warm enough

C of the danger of suffocation

D they are more difficult to keep clean

4 For sleeping, a baby

A needs a hard pillow

B needs a soft pillow

C needs a pillow under the mattress

D does not need a pillow

5 Bouncing cradles or rockers

A can be used for sleeping

B can be placed on a table

C should be placed on the floor

D are suitable for babies over 6 months of age

6 Two reaons why baby nests can be dangerous for babies are:

i ....

ii ....

7 Two essential safety features for baby chairs are:

i ....

ii ....

8 Baby bouncers and exercisers are suitable for:

A babies under 6 months

B babies over 6 months

C babies who are starting to stand

D babies who can walk

9 A safety harness for a pushchair needs:

A a waist strap

B waist and shoulder straps

C waist and crotch straps

D waist, shoulder and crotch straps

10 Consumer law gives certain rights to:

A customers

B users

C sellers

D customers, users and sellers

11 Three safety features for pushchairs and prams are:

i ....

ii ....

iii ....

1 To prevent the baby's head from being caught between the bars of the cot, the bars should be **45–65 mm apart**.

2 To prevent the baby's arms and legs from being trapped in the gap around the mattress, the gap should be no more than **40 mm**.

3 Duvets are not recommended for babies because **of the danger of suffocation**.

4 A baby **does not need a pillow** for sleeping. It is safer without one because of the danger of suffocation.

5 Bouncing cradles or rockers **should be placed on the floor**.

6 Baby nests can be dangerous when used for sleeping because:
  i   they may cause **suffocation**
  ii the baby may become **overhot**.

7 Baby chairs must:
  i   **be stable / have a broad base / not topple over**
  ii **have a safety harness**.

8 Baby bouncers and exercisers are suitable for babies **who are starting to stand**. They should stop being used as soon as the baby can walk unaided.

9 A safety harness for a pushchair needs **waist, shoulder and crotch straps**.

10 Consumer law gives certain rights to **customers** (consumers).

11 Safety features for pushchairs and prams are:
efficient brakes / be stable / do not topple over / have anchor points for a safety harness / a basket which fits underneath

Total number of marks	15
First time score	....
Score after revision	....

SECTION 4 DEVELOPMENT

CONTENTS

1 Each child is a unique person because each:
 A has a different set of genes
 B grows up in a different environment
 C has a different health record
 D has different genes, environment and health record

2 A child's environment means:
 A parks and gardens
 B all the surrounding conditions
 C the countryside
 D weather conditions

3 Identical twins have exactly the same:
 A genes
 B environment
 C health record
 D genes, environment and health record

4 Identical twins differ because of differences in their:
 A genes and environment
 B environment and health record
 C health record and genes
 D genes, environment and health record

5 Sort these environmental factors into those you consider to have a positive or a negative effect on growth and development:

being loved	being ignored	never being taken on outings
being listened to	being given over-strict	being cuddled and hugged
being spoilt	discipline	having companions to play
being over-protected	being given sufficient	with
receiving plenty of praise	discipline	having few toys or books in
being taken for outings	having toys and books	the home
being constantly criticised	being over-fussy about	being over-fussy about
being kept clean	tidyness	cleanliness
being played with	being regarded as a nuisance	

Positive effects on growth and development:

i ....

ii ....

iii ....

iv ....

v ....

vi ....

vii ....

viii ....

ix ....

x ....

Negative effects on growth and development:

i ....

ii ....

iii ....

iv ....

v ....

vi ....

vii ....

viii ....

ix ....

x ....

6 Babies gradually become aware of their name, body, age, family and home. This is known as their:
 A self-discipline
 B self-image
 C self-esteem
 D self-respect

7 Tick which of these you consider children should have experienced or learned by the time they are grown up:
 i how to give and receive love
 ii self-discipline
 iii success
 iv failure

1 Each child is a unique person because each **has different genes, environment and health record.**

2 A child's environment means **all the surrounding conditions** in which the child grows up. Besides including gardens, parks and the countryside, it also includes the conditions at home, the family's attitude towards education and the cultural life of the country.

3 Identical twins have exactly the same **genes**.

4 Identical twins differ because of differences in their **environment and health record.** For example, there will be differences in birthweights, accidents, illnesses and friends.

5

Positive effects on growth and development:	Negative effects on growth and development:
being loved	being spoilt
being listened to	being over-protected
being played with	being constantly criticised
receiving plenty of praise	being ignored
being taken for outings	being given over-strict discipline
being kept clean	being regarded as a nuisance
being cuddled and hugged	never being taken on outings
being given sufficient discipline	being over-fussy about tidyness
having toys and books	being over-fussy about cleanliness
having companions to play with	having few toys or books in the home

6 Babies gradually become aware of their name, body, age, family and home. This is known as their **self-image**.

7 By the time they are grown up children should have experienced or learned:

i   how to give and receive love   ✓
ii self-discipline   ✓
iii success   ✓
iv failure   ✓

Learning to cope with both success and failure is important as both are part of life. Being successful enhances self-esteem. Being unable to cope with failure can lower self-esteem.

Total number of marks   29
First time score   ....
Score after revision   ....

1 Genetics is the study of:
A dominant and recessive genes
B inherited disease
C the behaviour of chromosomes
D genes and their effects

2 Each gene contains a code which affects:
A a particular characteristic
B several characteristics
C growth
D development

3 Each chromosome contains:
A about a hundred genes
B several hundred genes
C about a thousand genes
D thousands of genes

4 The usual number of chromosomes in each cell is:
A 22
B 23
C 44
D 46

5 The number of chromosomes in each sex cell is:
A 22
B 23
C 44
D 46

6 Complete the diagram of fertilisation by using Y to represent the male sex chromosome, and X for the female sex chromosome.

7 Are uniovular twins:
A fraternal twins
B binovular twins
C identical twins
D non-identical twins?

8 The number of chromosomes in the body cells of a person with Down's syndrome is:
A 44
B 45
C 46
D 47

9 In which disease does very thick mucus clog the lungs?
A cystic fibrosis
B haemophilia
C sickle cell anaemia
D muscular dystrophy

10.In which disease is the blood unable to clot properly?
A cystic fibrosis
B haemophilia
C sickle cell anaemia
D muscular dystrophy

11 Which disease is caused by abnormal red cells?
A cystic fibrosis
B haemophilia
C sickle cell anaemia
D muscular dystrophy

12 Which disease makes movement difficult?
A cystic fibrosis
B haemophilia
C sickle cell anaemia
D muscular dystrophy

13 Which two inherited diseases occur only in boys?
A cystic fibrosis and haemophilia
B haemophilia and sickle cell anaemia
C sickle cell anaemia and Duchenne muscular dystrophy
D Duchenne muscular dystrophy and haemophilia

14 If a child inherits a dominant gene for black hair from one parent and a recessive gene for blonde hair from the other parent, the child will have:
A black hair
B brown hair
C blond hair
D auburn hair

1 Genetics is the study of **genes and their effects**.

2 Each gene contains a code which affects **a particular characteristic**.

3 Each chromosome contains **thousands of genes**.

4 The usual number of chromosomes in each cell is **46**.

5 The number of chromosomes in each sex cell is **23**.

6

Y + X = XY = boy

X + X = XX = girl

Diagram of fertilisation

(6 marks)

7 Uniovular twins are **identical twins**.

8 The number of chromosomes in the body cells of a person with Down's syndrome is **47** instead of the usual 46.

9 Very thick mucus clogs the lungs in people with **cystic fibrosis**.

10.The blood is unable to clot properly in people with **haemophilia**.

11 Abnormal red cells are found in people with **sickle cell anaemia**. The red cells change to a sickle shape when there is a shortage of oxygen.

12 Movements are difficult in people with **muscular dystrophy** because of weakness of the muscles.

13 Duchenne muscular dystrophy and haemophilia are inherited only by boys. Females can be carriers of the disease.

14 The child will have **black hair** because the gene for black hair is dominant to the recessive (weaker) gene for blond hair, and masks its effect.

Total number of marks	19
First time score	....
Score after revision	....

1 The most important factor controlling a child's growth in height is:
  A food intake
  B climate – warm or cold
  C the child's genes
  D the environment

2 Potential height is the:
  A average height of children of the same age
  B a child's final height
  C maximum height of children of the same age
  D maximum height that a child can reach

The weights of three boys in kilograms (kg)			
	Tom	Dick	Harry
Birth	2	3	4
1 year	8	9	11
2 years	11	12	13.5
3 years	13.5	13	16
4 years	16	14.5	18
5 years	18	15	22
6 years	20	17	25
7 years	23.5	19	28
8 years	25	20.5	32

5 On the weight chart, plot a graph of the weight of each of the boys above (hint: use a different colour for each boy, and label with the boy's name).

6 In which year did all the boys have the greatest increase in weight? ....

7 Which boy:
  i   was preterm? ....
  ii   had the heaviest birthweight? ....

3 Development is the process of:
  A becoming taller
  B learning new skills
  C becoming heavier
  D the process of growing

4 The 50th percentile on growth charts is the:
  A average growth rate for the age group
  B the growth rate of 50 children
  C the growth rate of 5000 children
  D the growth rate of half the children measured

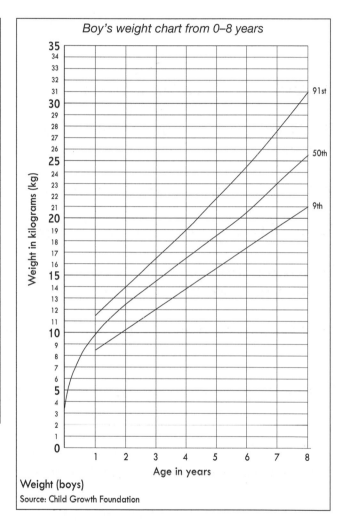

Boy's weight chart from 0–8 years

Weight (boys)
Source: Child Growth Foundation

8 Assuming that all the boys are of average height for their age, which boy:
  i   could be overweight? ....
  ii   could be failing to thrive? ....
  iii was closest to the average weight from 3–8 years? ....

1 The most important factor controlling a child's growth in height is **the child's genes**.

2 Potential height is the **maximum height that a child can reach** and depends on the genes which were inherited.

3 Development is the process of **learning new skills**.

4 The 50th percentile on growth charts is the **average rate for the age group**.

5

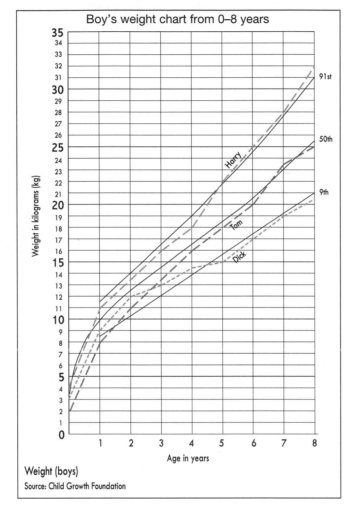

Weight (boys)
Source: Child Growth Foundation

(marks out of 3 for the accuracy of each graph, making a total of 9 marks)

6 The greatest increase in weight was during the **first year**. On average, a baby trebles its birthweight in the first year.

7 i   **Tom** was preterm. His birthweight was below 2.5 kg.
    ii   **Harry** had the heaviest birthweight.

8 i   **Harry**'s weight increased greatly above the average.
    ii   **Dick** could be failing to thrive as his weight was well below the average from 3 years onwards.
    iii   **Tom**'s weight was closest to the average from 3–8 years.

Total number of marks	19
First time score	....
Score after revision	....

1 Motor skills require coordination between:
A muscles and hands
B brain and muscles
C hands and nerves
D nerves and brain

2 An example of a gross motor skill is:
A kicking a ball
B doing up buttons
C using a knife and fork
D drawing a picture

3 A fine manipulative skill is:
A walking
B running
C kicking
D writing

4 Lying in the prone position is:
A lying on the back
B lying on the right side
C lying on the left side
D lying on the stomach

5 Which is *not* a main benefit of swimming?
A develops muscles and coordination
B improves breathing
C is an important safety skill
D development of manipulative skills

6 Who will be the most suitable person to give swimming lessons to children with special needs?
A physiologist
B physician
C psychiatrist
D physiotherapist

7 The average age at which babies can walk on their own is:
A 13 months
B 15 months
C 18 months
D 2 years

8 By what age can babies roll off the bed?
A 4 months
B 5 months
C 6 months
D 7 months

9 It is necessary to support a newborn baby's head because:
A it might fall backwards too far
B the top of the skull is delicate
C the brain is very delicate
D the neck muscles are very weak

10 People who are ambidextrous
A can kick a ball with either foot
B use different hands for different activities
C learn to ride a bicycle without difficulty
D can use both hands with equal ease

11 By what age should it be obvious if a child is right-handed or left-handed?
A 2 years
B 3 years
C 4 years
D 5 years

12 Use these statements to complete the sentences below:

warm water encourages painful joints to move   firms up floppy muscles

encourages concentration and perseverance   relaxes tight muscles

Swimming is beneficial for children with

i   arthritis because the...

ii   cerebral palsy because it...

iii learning difficulties because it...

iv Down's syndrome because it..

      and... (2 answers for question iv)

1 Motor skills require coordination between **brain and muscles**.

2 An example of a gross motor skill is **kicking a ball**. Gross motor skills use the large muscles.

3 A fine manipulative skill is **writing** because it requires precise use of the hands and fingers.

4 Lying in the prone position is **lying on the stomach**.

5 **Development of manipulative skills** is *not* a main benefit of swimming because the fine manipulative skills of the hands are not required.

6 A qualified **physiotherapist** is the most suitable person to give swimming lessons to children with special needs.

7 The average age at which babies first walk on their own is **13 months**.

8 When babies are able to roll over from their back onto their front, at the age of about **6 months**, they can easily roll off a bed.

9 It is necessary to support a newborn baby's head because **the neck muscles are very weak**.

10 Ambidextrous people **can use both hands with equal ease**.

11 By **4 years** of age should it be obvious if a child is right-handed or left-handed.

12 Swimming is beneficial for children with
   i   arthritis because the **warm water encourages painful joints to move**
   iii cerebral palsy because it **relaxes tight muscles**
   iii learning difficulties because it **encourages concentration and perseverance**
   iv Down's syndrome because it **firms up floppy muscles** and **encourages concentration and perseverance**.

Total number of marks	16
First time score	....
Score after revision	....

1 Label parts i–iv of the eye using the labels listed below (hint: the number of dashes in each label equals the number of letters in the answer):
iris
pupil
eyelid
white of the eye

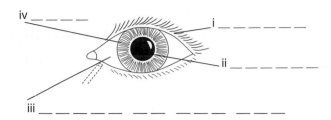

2 Label parts v–ix of the section through the eye using the labels listed below:
lens
retina
cornea (front of eye)
optic nerve
conjunctiva

3 Name the part of the eye which:

i   is a different colour in different people ....

ii   is a hole which lets the light through ....

iii if infected, causes conjunctivitis ....

iv   on which a stye may develop ....

v   if deeply scratched can damage eyesight ....

vi   contains the light-sensitive cells ....

4 Short sight means:
   A close objects cannot be seen clearly
   B things look blurred
   C distant objects cannot be seen clearly
   D the eyes look in different directions

5 Long sight means:
   A close objects cannot be seen clearly
   B things look blurred
   C distant objects cannot be seen clearly
   D the eyes look in different directions

6 Squint means:
   A close objects cannot be seen clearly
   B things look blurred
   C distant objects cannot be seen clearly
   D the eyes look in different directions

7 Astigmatism means:
   A close objects cannot be seen clearly
   B things look blurred
   C distant objects cannot be seen clearly
   D the eyes look in different directions

8 Newborn babies
   A can see nothing at all
   B are dimly aware of light
   C can see clearly
   D are very short-sighted

9 Short sight often develops at the age of:
   A 6–10 years
   B 4–8 years
   C 2–6 years
   D 6–8 years

10 Short sight or long sight:
   A gets worse if not treated
   B interferes with school work
   C makes things look crooked
   D encourages eye infections

11 Blind children:
   A can see nothing at all
   B usually have a little sight
   C can see in the dark
   D are colour blind

1 i   eyelid
   ii   pupil
   iii   white of the eye
   iv   iris

2 v   retina
   vi   optic nerve
   vii   conjunctiva
   viii lens
   ix   cornea

3 i   The **iris** is a different colour in different people.
   ii   The **pupil** is a hole which lets the light through.
   iii   If the **conjunctiva** is infected it causes conjunctivitis.
   iv   A stye develops on the **eyelid**.
   v   If the **cornea** is deeply scratched it may leave a scar on the eyeball.
   vi   The **retina** contains the light-sensitive cells.

4 Short sight means **distant objects cannot be seen clearly**.

5 Long sight means **close objects canot be seen clearly**.

6 Squint means **the eyes look in different directions**.

7 Astigmatism means **things look blurred**. Many people with this condition are not aware of it.

8 Newborn babies **are very short-sighted**. This condition gradually disappears as the eyes develop.

9 Short sight develops most often between the ages of **6 and 10 years**.

10 Short sight or long sight in a child needs to be detected as soon as possible because it will **interfere with school work** and, if not corrected by glasses, the child may be labelled restless, slow or lazy.

11 Blind children **usually have a little sight** but not enough to perform any task for which eyesight is essential.

Total number of marks	23
First time score	....
Score after revision	....

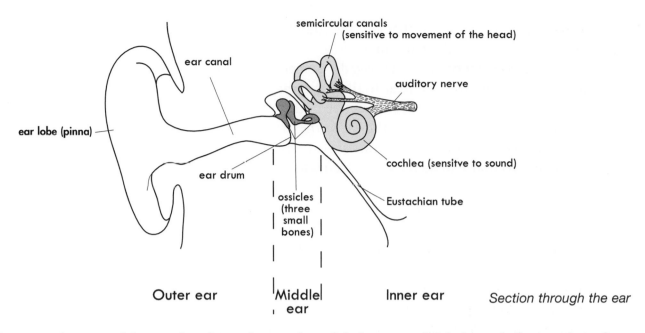

Section through the ear

1 Name the part of the ear that (hint: the number of dashes in each label equals the number of letters in the answer):

i   is visible and collects sound waves __ __ __   __ __ __ __ __

ii   produces wax __ __ __   __ __ __ __ __ __

iii   is easily damaged if something is poked into the ear   __ __ __   __ __ __ __ __

iv   link the outer ear with the inner ear __ __ __ __ __ __ __ __

v   contains the cells sensitive to the effects of sound __ __ __ __ __ __ __ __

vi   connects the ear to the brain __ __ __ __ __ __ __ __   __ __ __ __ __

vii links the middle ear with the throat __ __ __ __ __ __ __ __ __ __   __ __ __ __

viii is concerned with the balance of the body __ __ __ __ __ __ __ __ __ __ __ __ __

__ __ __ __ __ __

2 The middle ear contains the:
A ossicles
B cochlea
C semicircular canals
D ear canal

3 The inner ear contains the:
A ear drum and ossicles
B ossicles and cochlea
C cochlea and semicircular canals
D pinna and ear canal

4 Until what age does a deaf baby gurgle and babble like babies who can hear?
A 1 month
B 3 months
C 6 months
D 9 months

5 'Glue ear' is caused by a build-up of sticky fluid in the:
A outer ear
B middle ear
C inner ear
D ear canal

6 The neonatal audiological screen test is carried out on:
A new babies
B older babies
C toddlers
D pre-school children

7 Most deaf children
A hear nothing at all
B hear some sounds but not others
C are permanently deaf
D are temporarily deaf

1 i   The visible part of the ear that collects sound waves is the **ear lobe** (pinna).

ii   Wax is produced in the **ear canal**.

iii The **ear drum** can be easily damaged if something is poked into the ear.

iv   The **ossicles** link the outer ear to the inner ear.

v   The **cochlea** contains the cells sensitive to the effects of sound.

vi   The **auditory nerve** connects the ear to the brain.

vii The **Eustachian tube** links the middle ear with the throat.

viii The **semicircular canals** are concerned with the balance of the body.

2 The middle ear contains the **ossicles**.

3 The inner ear contains the **cochlea and semicircular canals**.

4 Until the age of **6 months** a deaf baby will use its voice to gurgle and babble in the same way as babies who can hear. The parents may not realise their baby has a hearing problem because the baby will respond to vibrations and loud noises.

5 'Glue ear' is caused by a build-up of sticky fluid in **the middle ear** following infection.

6 The neonatal audiological screen test is carried out on **new babies** (neo = new; natal = birth).

7 Most deaf children **hear some sounds but not others** so they cannot make sense of what they hear.

Total number of marks	14
First time score	....
Score after revision	....

1 Non-verbal communication means communicating:
A by email
B by letter
C without speaking
D by singing

2 Children learn to talk by:
A watching television
B listening to the radio
C copying sounds made by adults
D copying other children

3 Stammering is:
A uncommon in young children
B very rare in young children
C a stage many children pass through
D a stage a few children pass through

4 The average age at which a child's speech is easy to understand is:
A 3 years
B 4 years
C 5 years
D 6 years

5 Place the contents of the speech 'bubbles' in the usual order in which a child learns to speak.

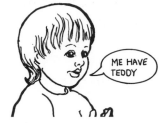
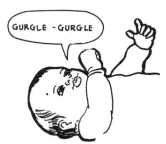
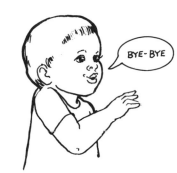
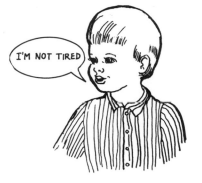
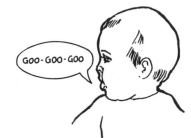
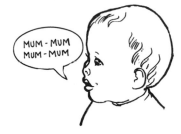
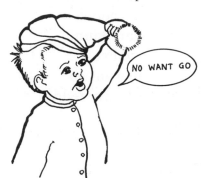
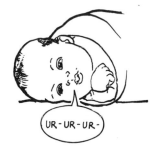

i ....
ii ....
iii ....
iv ....
v ....
vi ....
vii ....
viii ....

1 Non-verbal communication means communicating **without speaking**, for example by using the voice, the hands or expression on the face.

2 Children learn to talk by **copying sounds made by adults**.

3 Stammering is **a stage many children pass through** as they learn to speak. For most children the stage is temporary and they pass through it quite quickly.

4 A child's speech is usually easy to understand by **4 years** of age as most of the basic rules of grammar have been aquired.

5 i   **ur-ur-ur**
   ii   **gurgle-gurgle**
   iii   **goo-goo-goo**
   iv   **mum-mum**
   v   **bye-bye**
   vi   **no want go**
   vii   **me have teddy**
   viii **I'm not tired**

Total number of marks	12
First time score	....
Score after revision	....

1 Babies show that they have an inborn need for the company of other people when they cry because they are:
A hungry
B unwell
C tired
D lonely

2 Social development is the process of:
A learning to live easily with other people
B the development of social services
C learning about other cultures and societies
D the development of a social life

3 By what age do babies become shy when they meet strangers?
A 3 months
B 6 months
C 9 months
D 1 year

4 Who has the main responsibility for teaching social skills to children?
A teachers
B parents and carers
C friends
D social workers

5 The usual age at which a child can understand and obey simple commands is:
A 1 year
B 2 years
C 3 years
D 5–7 years

6 The usual age at which a child defends his possessions is:
A 2 years
B 3 years
C 4 years
D 5–7 years

6 The usual age at which a child understands the need for rules for fair play is:
A 2 years
B 3 years
C 4 years
D 5–7 years

8 The usual age at which a child understands sharing is:
A 2 years
B 3 years
C 4 years
D 5–7 years

9 Sort these social skills into two groups, good and poor:
stealing   always arguing   inoffensive eating habits
being able to share   being able to accept rules   never saying 'thank you'

Good social skills:

i ....

ii ....

iii ....

Poor social skills:

i ....

ii ....

iii ....

10 Identify the different stages of social play:
parallel play   joining-in play
looking-on play   co-operative play

iii ....

i ....

ii ....

iv ....

1 Babies show that they have an inborn need for the company of other people when they cry because they are **lonely**.

2 Social development is the process of **learning to live easily with other people**.

3 When about **9 months** old, babies often become shy when they meet strangers.

4 The main responsibility for teaching social skills to children is with **parents and carers**.

5 The usual age at which a child can understand and obey simple commands is **1 year**.

6 The usual age at which a child defends his possessions with determination is **2 years**.

7 The usual age at which a child understands the need for rules for fair play is **5–7 years**.

8 The usual age at which a child understands sharing is **3 years**.

9 Good social skills:
   i   **being able to share**
   ii   **beng able to accept rules**
   iii **inoffensive eating habits**

  Poor social skills:
   i   **stealing**
   ii   **always arguing**
   iii **never saying 'thank you'**

10 i   **joining-in play**
   ii   **parallel play**
   iii **looking-on play**
   iv **co-operative play**

Total number of marks	18
First time score	....
Score after revision	....

1 Emotions are:
A thoughts
B ideas
C feelings
D actions

2 Emotional development is the development of the ability to:
A recognise and control feelings
B remain calm
C be sensitive to other people
D be happy

3 Bonds of attachment are:
A strong feelings of affection
B one person's dependence on another
C the need for someone to depend on
D feelings of being tied to another person

4 Bonds of attachment are linked with feelings of:
A discipline and security
B comfort and security
C security and shyness
D discipline and shyness

5 Self-esteem means:
A being self-reliant
B having lots of self-confidence
C being very independent
D valuing yourself as a person

6 The main influence in helping a child to develop self-control is:
A the child's state of health
B training received from adults
C playing with other children
D an inborn knowledge

7 Children who often try too hard to please may:
A be self-confident
B have a low self-image
C have low self-control
D be self-reliant

8 Which action does *not* encourage a child's self-esteem?
A praise for what the child can do
B giving the child choices
C encouraging a child to express ideas
D criticism of what the child is unable to do

9 Lack of love makes a child feel:
A unhappy and insecure
B unhappy but secure
C secure but unhappy
D happy and sad

10 'Smother' love may prevent a child from:
A being over-protected
B playing without constant interference
C being under protected
D learning to become independent

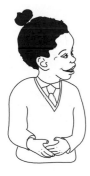

11 Sort the statements into those which help and those which hinder the development of self-esteem.

being valued by family   feeling unappreciated
feeling worthless   being supported
constant criticism   being valued by friends
being encouraged   getting into trouble at school
getting into trouble at home   being praised

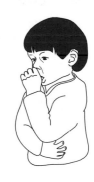

Olive develops self-esteem when she is:

i ....

ii ....

iii ....

iv ....

v ....

Oliver's low self-esteem comes from:

i ....

ii ....

iii ....

iv ....

v ....

1 Emotions are **feelings**, such as excitement, fear and affection.

2 Emotional development is the development of the ability to **recognise and control feelings**.

3 Bonds of attachment are **strong feelings of affection**.

4 Bonds of attachment are linked with feelings of **comfort and security**.

5 Self-esteem means **valuing yourself as a person**.

6 The main influence in helping a child to develop self-control is **training received from adults**.

7 Children who often try too hard to please may **have a low self-image**.

8 A child's self-esteem is not encouraged by **criticism of what the child is unable to do**.

9 Lack of love makes a child feel **unhappy and insecure**.

10 'Smother' love may prevent a child from **learning to become independent**.

11 Olive is helped to develop self-esteem when she is:
   i   **valued by family**
   ii   **encouraged**
   iii   **supported by family and friends**
   iv   **valued by friends**
   v   **praised**

Oliver's low self-esteem comes from:
   i   **feeling worthless**
   ii   **constant criticism**
   iii   **getting into trouble at home**
   iv   **feeling unappreciated**
   v   **getting into trouble at school**

Total number of marks	20
First time score	....
Score after revision	....

moves arms, legs and head

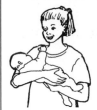

very shortsighted

does not play

hands usually closed

comforted by being held close

Newborn

---

plays with fingers

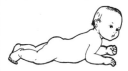

hands usually open

smiles at people

can see things nearby

some head control

3 months

---

can see things further away

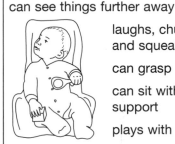

laughs, chuckles and squeals

can grasp a rattle

can sit with support

plays with rattles

6 months

---

recognises people at a distance

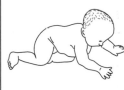

enjoys putting things in and out of boxes

opens hands to drop things

tries to crawl

shy with strangers

9 months

---

eyes follow rapidly moving objects

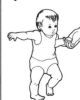

enjoys looking at picture books

points to things

understands the meaning of 'No'

begins to walk

1 year

Each child is an individual and the age at which normal children sit, walk, talk and so on varies enormously. The information given here shows the average age at which a particular stage of development takes place. Use the information accompanying the pictures to complete the chart below.

Body movements

Newborn

3 months

6 months

9 months

1 year

Using the hands

Newborn

3 months

6 months

9 months

1 year

Eyes

Newborn

3 months

6 months

9 months

1 year

Play

Newborn

3 months

6 months

9 months

1 year

Behaviour

Newborn

3 months

6 months

9 months

1 year

Body movements
Newborn	moves arms, legs and head
3 months	some head control
6 months	can sit with support
9 months	tries to crawl
1 year	begins to walk

Using the hands
Newborn	hands usually closed
3 months	hands usually open
6 months	can grasp a rattle
9 months	opens hands to drop things
1 year	points to things

Eyes
Newborn	very short-sighted
3 months	can see things nearby
6 months	can see things further away
9 months	recognises people at a distance
1 year	eyes follow rapidly moving objects

Play
Newborn	does not play
3 months	plays with fingers
6 months	plays with rattles
9 months	enjoys putting things in and out of boxes
1 year	enjoys looking at picture books

Behaviour
Newborn	comforted by being held close
3 months	smiles at people
6 months	laughs, chuckles and squeals
9 months	shy with strangers
1 year	understands the meaning of 'No'

Total number of marks	25
First time score	....
Score after revision	....

enjoys playing with bricks

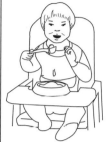

likes to 'help' adults

can feed himself

can walk upstairs

18 months

---

can walk up and down stairs

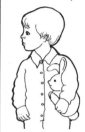

turns door handles

the 'No' stage

sees as clearly as an adult

enjoys playing with balls

2 years

---

can walk on tiptoe

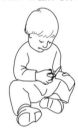

knows red and yellow

uses scissors

asks many questions

enjoys drawing and painting

3 years

---

can hop

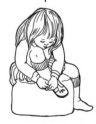

knows blue and green

can dress and undress alone

good bladder control

enjoys dressing-up games

4 years

---

is more independent

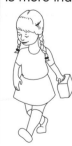

can use a knife and fork

can skip

enjoys computer games

knows most colours

5 years

Use the information accompanying the different stages of development to complete the chart below, remembering that the information given refers to the average attainment. Some children will be ahead of, and others behind, the average for that age stage.

Body movements

18 months

2 years

3 years

4 years

5 years

Using the hands

18 months

2 years

3 years

4 years

5 years

Eyes

2 years

3 years

4 years

5 years

Play

18 months

2 years

3 years

4 years

5 years

Behaviour

18 months

2 years

3 years

4 years

5 years

Body movements

18 months	can walk upstairs
2 years	can walk up and down stairs
3 years	can walk on tiptoe
4 years	can hop
5 years	can skip

Using the hands

18 months	can feed himself
2 years	turns door handles
3 years	uses scissors
4 years	can dress and undress alone
5 years	can use a knife and fork

Eyes

2 years	sees as clearly as an adult
3 years	knows red and yellow
4 years	knows blue and green
5 years	knows most colours

Play

18 months	enjoys playing with bricks
2 years	enjoys playing with balls
3 years	enjoys drawing and painting
4 years	enjoys dressing-up games
5 years	enjoys computer games

Behaviour

18 months	likes to 'help' adults
2 years	the 'No' stage
3 years	asks many questions
4 years	good bladder control
5 years	is more independent

Total number of marks	24
First time score	....
Score after revision	....

1 Chose three of the statements below that explain why children need discipline:
  • to teach them what is safe and unsafe
  • to make them do as they are told
  • so that they do not embarrass their parents
  • so that they are a credit to their parents
  • to learn that there are consequences for misbehaviour
  • to help them to learn to control their own behaviour (learn self-control)

i ....

ii ....

iii...

2 Discipline should begin:
  A soon after birth
  B at about six months of age
  C when the child is able to understand what is required
  D when the child is ready for school

3 Good discipline involves:
  A correction and criticism
  B obedience and good manners
  C slapping when necessary
  D setting clear, reasonable limits for behaviour

4 Write the statements in the appropriate boxes below (two per box).

    weak   consistent   demands too much
    fair   unreasonable   inconsistent

Good discipline:	**Poor discipline:**	**Excessive discipline:**
i	i	i ....
ii	ii	ii ....

5 Draw lines to match each of the statements below with its explanation.
  Ways of encouraging good behaviour:

  i   Set a good example   children cannot be forced to eat or sleep
  ii   Praise rather than criticise   'NO' means 'NO'
  iii Be reasonable in what is expected   children imitate adults
  iv   Be consistent   children need time to learn
  v   Mean what you say   it helps children to learn to say sorry
  vi   Avoid battles which cannot be won   praise is more effective than criticism
  vii Say sorry for your own poor behaviour rules which are made should be kept

1 Children need discipline (answers can be in any order):
   i **to teach them what is safe and unsafe**
   ii **to learn that there are consequences for misbehaviour**
   iii **to help them to learn to control their own behaviour (i.e. learn self-control).**

2 Discipline should begin **when the child is able to understand what is required**.

3 Good discipline involves **setting clear, reasonable limits for behaviour** so that the child knows what is expected.

4 Good discipline:
   i **fair**
   ii **consistent**

Poor discipline:
   i **weak**
   ii **inconsistent**

Excessive discipline:
   i **unreasonable**
   ii **demands too much**

5 Ways of encouraging good behaviour:
   i Set a good example because **children imitate adults**.
   ii Praise rather than criticise because **praise is more effective than criticism** in the training of children.
   iii Be reasonable in what is expected because **children need time to learn**.
   iv Be consistent because **rules which are made should be kept**.
   v Mean what you say – **'NO' means 'NO'**.
   vi Avoid battles which cannot be won – **children cannot be forced to eat or sleep**.
   vii Say sorry for poor behaviour because **it helps children to learn to say sorry**.

Total number of marks	18
First time score	....
Score after revision	....

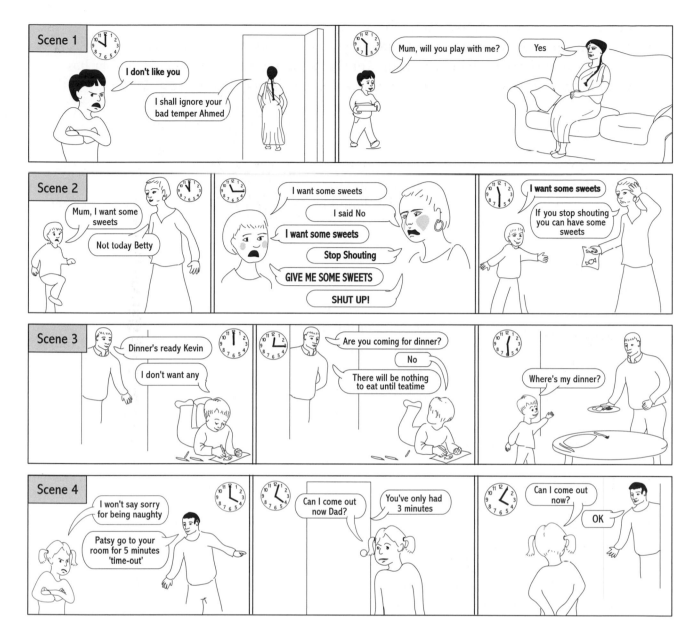

1 On a spare piece of paper and in your own words, describe what is happening in scenes 1–4 (10 marks per scene).

2 In which scene was the child being taught to shout to get what he/she wants?
 A Scene 1
 B Scene 2
 C Scene 3
 D Scene 4

3 In which scenes does the parent *not* mean what he/she says?
 A Scenes 1 and 2   C Scenes 2 and 4
 B Scenes 2 and 3   D Scenes 1 and 4

4 In which scenes does the parent mean what he/she says?
 A Scenes 1 and 2   C Scenes 3 and 4
 B Scenes 2 and 3   D Scenes 1 and 4

5 Knowing how to behave in an acceptable manner
 A is inborn in children
 B is taught to children by adults
 C is something they learn for themselves
 D can be picked up from television

6 Which scenes help a child in learning to behave in a socially acceptable manner?
 A Scenes 1 and 2   C Scenes 2 and 4
 B Scenes 2 and 3   D Scenes 1 and 4

Scene 1

Ahmed (1) was in a bad temper (1) and shouting (1) at his mother (1). His mother walks out of the room (1) and ignores his bad behaviour. (1) Half an hour later (1) Ahmed's temper has improved / he is now in a happier frame of mind (1) and asks (1) his mother (1) to play with him (1), and she agrees.

(10 marks maximum)

Scene 2

Betty (1) is shouting (1) at her mother (1) asking for sweets (1). Her mother (1) shouts back (1) telling Betty (1) to 'shut up' (1). Half an hour later (1) when Betty demands / shouts for sweets again (1), her mother (1) gives them (1) to her.

(10 marks maximum)

Scene 3

Dad (1) tells Kevin (1) that his dinner is ready (1). Kevin says he does not want any (1). Fifteen minutes later (1) Kevin was asked if he was coming for his dinner (1), and said 'No' (1). His dad then told him (1) there will be nothing to eat until tea-time (1). Fifteen minutes later (1), when Kevin wanted his dinner (1), his dad gave it to him (1).

(10 marks maximum)

Scene 4

Patsy (1) wouldn't say sorry (1) and her dad (1) told her to go to her room (1) for five minutes (1) for 'time out' (1). After three minutes (1) Patsy asked if she could come out (1). She was told 'No' (1) as she had only been in her room for three minutes (1). When the five minutes was up (1), Patsy asked if she could come out (1) and her dad said OK (1).

(10 marks maximum)

2   In **scene 2** Betty was being taught to shout to get what she wants.

3   In **scene 1 and scene 4** the parent means what he/she says.

4   In **scene 2 and scene 3** the parent does not mean what he/she says.

5   Knowing how to behave in an acceptable manner **is taught to children by adults**.

6   **Scene 1 and scene 4** help a child in learning to behave in a socially acceptable manner.

Total number of marks	45
First time score	....
Score after revision	....

1 Use the words to complete the sentences below:

action   bladder   bowel   faeces   muscles   motion   stools   urine

i   Liquid waste from the body is stored in the __ __ __ __ __ __ __ .

ii Liquid waste is called __ __ __ __ __ .

iii Solid waste matter is stored in the __ __ __ __ __ .

iv The technical name for the solid waste matter is __ __ __ __ __ __ .

v   Faeces may be called __ __ __ __ __ __ , the __ __ __ __ __ __ or bowel __ __ __ __ __ __ .

vi A child has to learn to control the __ __ __ __ __ __ __ of the bladder and bowel.

2 Place these stages of learning to control the bladder in the correct order:

the child is able to tell someone in time to be put on the potty
the child knows when she is about to wet her nappy
the child indicates when she has a wet nappy
the child knows when she is wetting her nappy

i   ....

ii ....

iii ....

iv ....

3 Starting to be able to control the bladder and bowel rarely happens before the age of:
A 9 months
B 1 year
C 15–18 months
D 18 months–2 years

4 Is bowel control likely to be learnt
A before bladder control
B at the same time as bladder control
C just after bladder control
D about a year after bladder control?

5 Who is likely to be potty-trained more quickly, the child
A who is made to sit on the potty
B who is worried about wetting her pants
C whose mother is obsessed by potty training
D who is given gentle encouragement to use the potty?

6 About how many children are still wetting the bed occasionally at the age of five?
A 1%
B 10%
C 20%
D 25%

1 i Liquid waste from the body is stored in the **bladder**.
    ii Liquid waste is called **urine**.
    iii Solid waste matter is stored in the **bowel**.
    iv The technical name for the solid waste matter is **faeces**.
    v Faeces may be called the **stools**, the **motion** or bowel **action**.
    vi A child has to learn to control the **muscles** of the bladder and bowel.

2 Stages of learning to control the bladder:
    i **the child indicates when she has a wet nappy**
    ii **the child knows when she is wetting her nappy**
    iii **the child knows when she is about to wet her nappy**
    iv **the child is able to tell someone in time to be put on the potty**.

3 Starting to learn to control the muscles which open the bladder and bowel rarely happens before the age of **15–18 months**, and often not until 2–3 years old.

4 Bowel control is likely to be learnt **before bladder control**.

5 The child who is likely to be potty-trained more quickly is the one **given gentle encouragement to use the potty**.

6 About **10%** of children are still wetting the bed occasionally at the age of five.

Total number of marks	16
First time score	....
Score after revision	....

1 Intellectual development is:
A increase in size of the brain
B being able to read easily
C development of the mind
D the number of exams taken

2 Intellectual development may also be known as:
A cognitive development
B emotional development
C physical development
D language development

3 How intelligent a child becomes depends mainly on:
A the child's genes
B the child's environment
C the child's genes and environment
D none of the above

4 Knowing the difference between right and wrong is:
A inborn in children
B mainly taught to children by adults
C something they learn for themselves
D picked up from television

5 Sort the conditions listed below into two groups – those which encourage intellectual development and those which hinder it:

listening to stories   bullying   having nothing of interest to do
poor eyesight   having questions answered   having adults to talk to and play with
deafness   frequent illness   frequent absences from school
exploring new places   having access to books   having opportunities to try new skills

Encourage development of the mind: **Hinder development of the mind:**

i...   i   ....

ii..   ii ....

iii...   iii ....

iv...   iv ....

v..   v   ....

vi...   vi ....

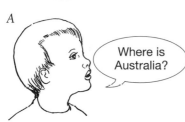

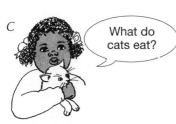

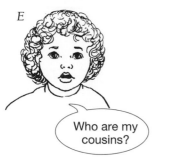

6 When children are able to talk, they start to ask questions. They do this:
A to get someone to pay attention to them
B for something to say
C to annoy their parents
D to make sense of their world

7 Which of these children (A–F) is learning about

i   people ....

ii places ....

ii time........................

iv plants ....

v   objects.....................

vi animals? ....

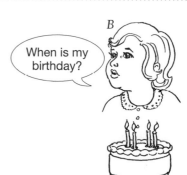

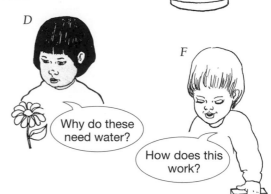

1 Intellectual development is **development of the mind**. The mind is the thinking part of the brain – the part used for recognising, reasoning, knowing and understanding.

2 Intellectual development may also be known as **cognitive development** (the process of acquiring knowledge).

3 How intelligent a child becomes depends mainly on **the child's genes and environment**.

4 Knowing the difference between right and wrong **is mainly taught to children by adults**.

5 Development of the mind is encouraged by:
listening to stories
exploring new places
having questions answered
having access to books
having adults to talk to and play with
having opportunities to try new skills

Development of the mind is hindered by:
poor eyesight
deafness
bullying
frequent illness
having nothing of interest to do
frequent absences from school

6 When children are able to talk, they start to ask questions. They do this **to make sense of their world**.

7 i   people   E
ii places   A
iii time   B
iv plants   D
v   objects   F
vi animals   C

Total number of marks	23
First time score	....
Score after revision	....

SECTION 5   EARLY CHILDHOOD

CONTENTS

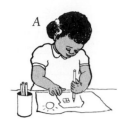 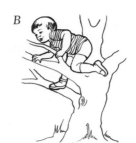 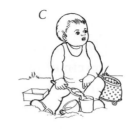 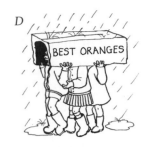

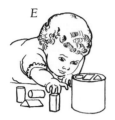 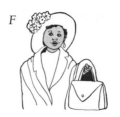

Descriptions:
finding out (e.g. about sand)
being active
making something original
pretend play
using the hands
children playing together

1 Complete the chart below by:
i identifying the types of play shown in A–F
ii adding a description for each from the list on the right

Type of play	Description	Drawing
Imaginative		
Manipulative		
Creative		
Discovery		
Physical		
Social		

1 Complete the chart above by:
i adding a description for each type of play from the box above
ii choosing one of the drawings A–F that best illustrates that type of play

2 Which type of play A–F:

i helps in speech development? ....

ii helps to develop gross motor skills? ....

iii involves role-play? ....

iv involves sharing? ....

v explores texture? ....

vi helps to develop fine motor skills?

........., ..., ... (3 answers)

3 Children play because:
A they are expected to do so
B they enjoy it
C it keeps them occupied
D adults tell them to

4 It is important to provide facilities to encourage children to play because:
A while they are playing they are learning
B it stops them annoying adults
C it keeps them occupied
D it gives them something to do

5 When an adult plays a game with a young child, should the adult
A tell the child what to do?
B correct the child when necessary?
C follow the child's lead?
D expect the child to follow the rules?

1

Type of play	Description	Drawing
Imaginative play	**pretend play**	F
Manipulative play	**using the hands**	E
Creative play	**making something original**	A
Discovery play	**finding out (e.g. about sand)**	C
Physical play	**being active**	B
Social play	**children playing together**	D

(12 marks)

2 Which type of play A–F
   i   helps in speech development   **D**
   ii helps to develop gross motor skills **B**
   iii involves role-play   **F**
   iv involves sharing   **D**
   v   explores texture   **C**
   vi helps to develop fine motor skills?   **A, C and E**

3 Children play because **they enjoy it**. They do not play when it is not enjoyable or if they are bored with the game.

4 It is important to provide facilities to encourage children to play because **while they are playing they are learning**.

5 A child will enjoy games with an adult when the adult **follows the child's lead**. Young children enjoy using their imagination, and have fun inventing their own rules.

Total number of marks   23
First time score   ....
Score after revision   ....

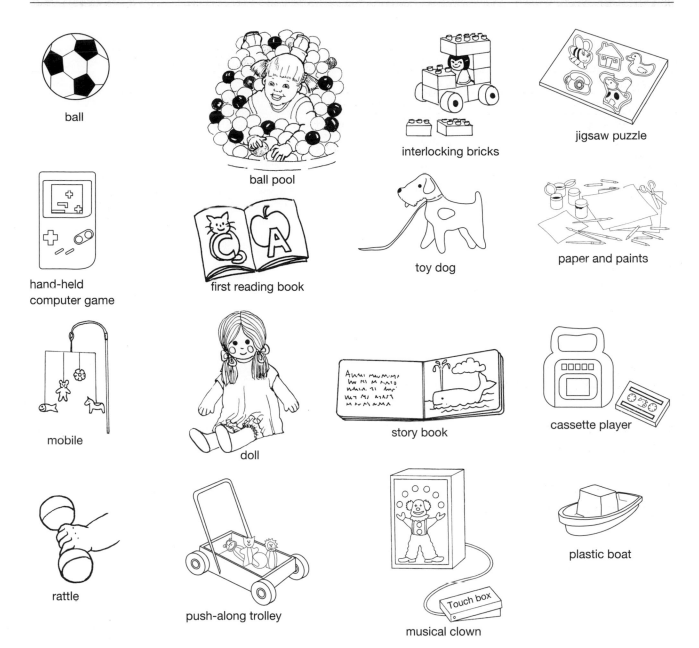

ball

ball pool

interlocking bricks

jigsaw puzzle

hand-held computer game

first reading book

toy dog

paper and paints

mobile

doll

story book

cassette player

rattle

push-along trolley

musical clown

Touch box

plastic boat

Choose the most suitable toy for each of the catagories below.

i   bathtime...

ii   a first toy...

iii   a pretend pet..

iv   active games..

v   fixing to a cot...

vi   an imaginary friend....................................

vii   matching things ....

viii   strengthening muscles................................

ix   creative activities.......................................

x   long car journeys ....

xi   learning the alphabet ....

xii   a child who can read..................................

xiii   building things..

xiv   a child who cannot grasp ....

xv   playing nursery rhymes...............................

xvi   learning to walk ....

A toy suitable for:

i	bathtime	**plastic boat**
ii	a first toy	**rattle**
iii	a pretend pet	**toy dog**
iv	active games	**ball**
v	fixing to a cot	**mobile**
vi	an imaginary friend	**doll**
vii	matching things	**jigsaw puzzle**
viii	strengthening muscles	**ball pool**
ix	creative activities	**paper and paints**
x	long car journeys	**hand-held computer game**
xi	learning the alphabet	**first reading book**
xii	a child who can read	**story book**
xiii	building things	**interlocking bricks**
xiv	a child who cannot grasp	**musical clown**
xv	playing nursery rhymes	**cassette player**
xvi	learning to walk	**push-along trolley**

Total number of marks	16
First time score	....
Score after revision	....

1 By what age are children able to hold markers and crayons?
A 12–18 months
B 18 months–2 years
C 2 years
D 3 years

2 By about which age has a child's imagination developed enough to start drawing pictures, e.g. a circle for a face?
A 12 months
B 18 months
C 2 years
D 3 years

3 The nine statements in this list describe the order of the stages in which children learn to draw.
1 Backwards and forwards scribble
2 Lifts crayon from the paper and makes lines
3 Scribbles in circles
4 Draws a circle for a face, with eyes, nose and mouth
5 Lines added around the face
6 Arms, legs and hair come from the face
7 Smaller circle below face for the body
8 Body has clothes and legs have feet
9 The drawing has people and other objects from the child's world

For each of the drawings:
i   identify the stage number
ii copy the statement to describe it.

Stage ....
....

Stage ....
....

Stage ....
....

Stage ....
....

Stage ....
....

Stage ....
....

Stage ....
....

Stage ....
....

Stage ....
....

1 Children are able to hold markers and crayons by about the age of **12–18 months**.

2 By about **2 years** of age a child's imagination has developed enough to start drawing pictures.

3

Stage **1**
Backwards and forwards scribble

Stage **2**
Lifts crayon from the paper and makes lines

Stage **3**
Scribbles in circles

Stage **4**
Draws a circle for a face, with eyes, nose, mouth

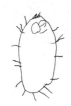
Stage **5**
Lines added around the face

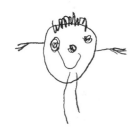
Stage **6**
Arms, legs and hair come from the face

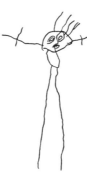
Stage **7**
Smaller circle below face for the body

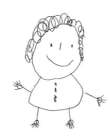
Stage **8**
Body has clothes and legs have feet

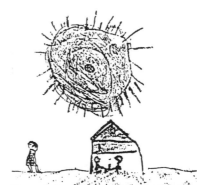
Stage **9**
The drawing has people and other objects from the child's world

(2 marks for each drawing: 1 for the correct stage and 1 for the correct description)

Total number of marks	20
First time score	....
Score after revision	....

Across

1 Sam can't read yet but he enjoys looking at these in his books (8)

6 Both boys and __ __ __ __ __ like exciting stories (5)

7 David has no-one to __ __ __ __ __ books with (5)

9 Jill __ __ __ __ __ __ with her left hand (6)

11 Children like stories read to them when they are __ __ __ (3)

12 This is used to write with (3)

13 When children __ __ __ __ older they learn to do joined-up writing (4)

14 Children have to be taught to read by adults, and __ __ __ _ to write (4)

17 Tracey __ __ learning her letters (2)

18 When dad reads a story, Cara can now __ __ __ __ __ __ the words in the book (6)

20 'Sing __ __ __ __ __ of sixpence' is a popular nursery rhyme (1, 4)

22 Derek likes to __ __ __ __ __ __ to his story tapes (6)

23 When the teacher reads a story, the children sit __ __ the floor (2)

Down

1 Jim knows that you must read from left to right across the __ __ __ __ (4)

2 Debby and her __ __ __ __ __ enjoy reading books together (5)

3 Amy gets __ __ __ __ __ when her reading is corrected too often (5)

4 Poor __ __ __ sight makes reading difficult (3)

5 Means 'word blindness' (8)

8 Letters __ __ __ __ together to make words (4)

9 These join together to make sentences (5)

10 T and i and n and a __ __ __ __ __ __ Tina (6)

14 Lana is a girl's name. Change the letters around to make a boy's name (4)

15 Jane will __ __ __ __ be ready to learn to read (4)

16 Celia has a bookshelf for her __ __ __ books

19 Sammy likes to cuddle close to his mum __ __ she reads to him (2)

21 George likes to __ __ to the library (2)

© Hodder Arnold 2005

¹P	I	²C	T	³U	R	⁴E	S		
A		A		P		Y			⁵D
⁶G	I	R	L	S		⁷E	N	⁸J	O	Y
E		E		E			O		S
	⁹W	R	I	T	E	¹⁰S		¹¹I	L	L
	O				¹²P	E	N		E
¹³G	R	O	W		E			X
	D		¹⁴A	L	¹⁵S	¹⁶O		I
¹⁷I	S		¹⁸F	O	L	L	O	W	A
	¹⁹A		²⁰A	S	O	N	²¹G
²²L	I	S	T	E	N		N		²³O	N

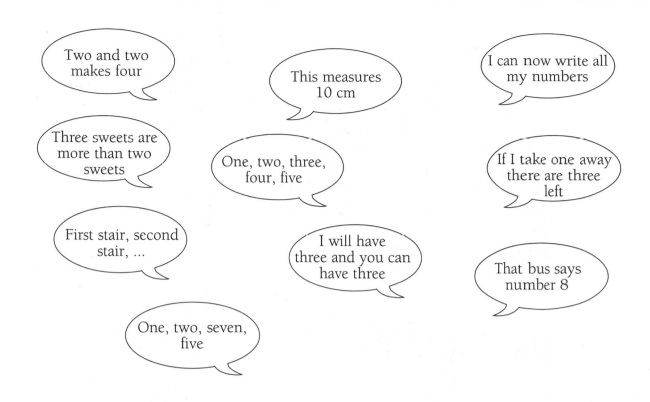

1 Write the words in each speech bubble against the appropriate stage in learning about numbers:

i Saying number words in any order ....

ii The correct order of the numbers ....

iii Understanding 'first', 'second', 'last' ....

iv Comparing numbers ....

v Recognising numbers ....

vi Writing numbers ....

vii Adding numbers together ....

viii Taking numbers away ....

ix Sharing ....

x Measuring ....

Which of the above stages correspond to these rhymes/songs for children?

2 One, two, buckle my shoe
Three, four, knock at the door

stage ....

3 Ten green bottles
Hanging on the wall
And if one green bottle
Should accidently fall
There'll be nine green bottles
Hanging on the wall

stage ....

1 Stages of learning about numbers:

  i   **One, two, seven, five**

  ii   **One, two, three, four, five**

  iii **First stair, second stair, ...**

  iv   **Three sweets are more than two sweets**

  v   **That bus says number 8**

  vi   **I can now write all my numbers**

  vii **Two and two makes four**

  viii **If I take one away there are three left**

  ix   **I will have three and you can have three**

  x   **This measures 10 cm**.

2 Stage **ii**

3 Stage **viii**

Total number of marks	12
First time score	....
Score after revision	....

1 From what age are babies aware of the soothing sounds of a lullaby?
A newborn
B 6 months
C 9 months
D 1 year

2 By what age do babies enjoy musical mobiles?
A newborn
B 3 months
C 9 months
D 1 year

3 By what age do babies enjoy joining in songs?
A 3 months
B 6 months
C 9 months
D 1 year

4 Is the game for children below designed for
A drama lessons
B keep fit lessons
C music lessons
D singing lessons?

5 These children are responding to changes in the music by using different actions. Label:

loud sounds
low notes
fast
slow
high notes
soft sounds

ii .... iii ....

iv ....

i ....

v ....

vi ....

Pitch   Volume   Tempo (speed)

6 Complete the titles of these popular songs for young children:

i   Pop goes the _ _ _ _ _ _

ii   _ _ _ _ _ Jacques

iii Incy Wincy _ _ _ _ _ _

iv   Sing a Song of _ _ _ _ _ _ _ _

v   Rock-a-Bye _ _ _ _ _

vi   _ _ _ _ _ _ Bridge is Falling Down

vii Ring-a-Ring of _ _ _ _ _ _

viii Polly, put the _ _ _ _ _ _ _ on

ix   _ _ _ _ _ _ _ and Lemons

x   Here we go Round the _ _ _ _ _ _ _ _ _ _ _ _ _

xi   Old _ _ _ _ _ _ _ _ _ _ _ had a Farm

xii Hot Cross _ _ _ _ _

xiii O Dear, What can the _ _ _ _ _ _ _ be

xiv Twinkle, Twinkle _ _ _ _ _ _ _ _ _ _ _ _ _

xv   Humpty _ _ _ _ _ _ _

xvi The Grand Old _ _ _ _ _ of _ _ _ _

7 Name one of the songs above that:

i   helps children to learn about noises made by animals...

ii   helps children to learn about places ....

iii is in a different language...

iv   is part of a game where children form a circle...

v   has particular actions to accompany the song...

1 **Newborn** babies are aware of the soothing sounds of a lullaby.

2 By **3 months** old babies enjoy musical mobiles.

3 By **1 year** old babies enjoy joining in songs, for example by clapping their hands.

4 The game shown for children is designed for **music lessons** to teach them about pitch, volume and tempo (speed).

5 i   **low notes**
   ii **high notes**
   iii **soft sounds**
   iv **loud sounds**
   v   **fast**
   vi **slow**

6 i   Pop goes the **Weasel**
   ii   **Frère** Jacques
   iii Incy Wincy **Spider**
   iv Sing a Song of **Sixpence**
   v   Rock-a-Bye **Baby**
   vi   **London** Bridge is Falling Down
   vii Ring-a-Ring of **Roses**
   viii Polly, put the **Kettle** on

   ix   **Oranges** and Lemons
   x   Here we go Round the **Mulberry Bush**
   xi   Old **MacDonald** had a Farm
   xii Hot Cross **Buns**
   xiii O Dear, What can the **Matter Be**
   xiv Twinkle, Twinkle **Little Star**
   xv Humpty **Dumpty**
   xvi The Grand Old **Duke** of **York**

7 i   **Old MacDonald had a Farm**
   ii   **London Bridge is Falling Down**
   iii **Frère Jacques**
   iv **Ring-a-Ring of Roses / Here we go Round the Mulberry Bush**
   v   **Oranges and Lemons / Incy Wincy Spider / Rock-a-Bye Baby / Ring-a-Ring of Roses / Twinkle Twinkle Little Star / The Grand Old Duke of York**.

Total number of marks	31
First time score	....
Score after revision	....

1 Some types of **behaviour common in young children** occur as they learn to behave in a socially acceptable way, challenging the rules as they do so, in an attempt to 'get their own way'.

Other types of behaviour are dangerous or abusive, and damaging to people or their property. These types of behaviour are regarded as **antisocial behaviour**.

In the boxes below, mark six types of **antisocial behaviour** with the letter 'A' and six types of **behaviour common in young children** with the letter 'B'.

☐ bullying   ☐ minor squabbles   ☐ verbal abuse and swearing
☐ pouting   ☐ starting fires   ☐ whining
☐ persistent hitting and biting   ☐ persistent stealing   ☐ smart talk
☐ making faces   ☐ temper tantrums   ☐ damaging property

2 Complete the wordsearch by finding the words above which have been underlined.

A	T	V	R	B	H	S	L	U	N	T	E	S	E	S	O
D	A	M	A	G	I	N	G	P	R	O	P	E	R	T	Y
E	N	G	R	O	T	C	S	A	D	X	O	L	J	A	E
U	T	Y	T	U	T	M	W	K	A	B	U	S	E	R	H
R	R	Z	E	A	I	C	E	A	T	P	T	I	N	T	R
R	U	N	N	I	N	G	A	W	A	Y	I	S	O	I	G
E	M	A	D	R	G	T	R	K	D	O	N	I	G	N	D
A	S	W	E	A	P	F	I	R	S	S	G	Q	U	G	L
I	L	E	D	O	V	U	N	G	A	M	B	X	W	F	E
B	U	L	L	Y	I	N	G	E	A	A	V	E	H	I	T
J	E	X	A	R	W	I	S	T	H	R	U	M	I	R	E
S	S	T	E	A	L	I	N	G	P	T	O	R	N	E	S
L	O	A	B	W	O	Y	E	S	C	T	L	I	I	S	K
Q	R	B	I	T	I	N	G	W	A	A	Y	U	N	A	P
U	S	E	E	K	T	O	P	M	T	L	E	S	G	A	Y
S	Q	U	A	B	B	L	E	S	P	K	V	A	W	T	H

1 [A] bullying   [A] persistent stealing
   [B] pouting   [B] temper tantrums
   [A] persistent hitting and biting   [A] verbal abuse and swearing
   [B] making faces   [B] whining
   [B] miner squabbles   [B] smart talk
   [A] starting fires   [A] damaging property

2 bullying   biting   stealing   swearing   damaging property
   pouting   squabbles   tantrums   whining
   hitting   starting fires abuse   smart talk

```
A  T  V  R  B  H  S  L  U  N  T  E  S  E  S  O
D  A  M  A  G  I  N  G  P  R  O  P  E  R  T  Y
E  N  G  R  O  T  C  S  A  D  X  O  L  J  A  E
U  T  Y  T  U  T  M  W  K  A  B  U  S  E  R  H
R  R  Z  E  A  I  C  E  A  T  P  T  I  N  T  R
R  U  N  N  I  N  G  A  W  A  Y  I  S  O  I  G
E  M  A  D  R  G  T  R  K  D  O  N  I  G  N  D
A  S  W  E  A  P  F  I  R  S  S  G  Q  U  G  L
I  L  E  D  O  V  U  N  G  A  M  B  X  W  F  E
B  U  L  L  Y  I  N  G  E  A  A  V  E  H  I  T
J  E  X  A  R  W  I  S  T  H  R  U  M  I  R  E
S  S  T  E  A  L  I  N  G  P  T  O  R  N  E  S
L  O  A  B  W  O  Y  E  S  C  T  L  I  I  S  K
Q  R  B  I  T  I  N  G  W  A  A  Y  U  N  A  P
U  S  E  E  K  T  O  P  M  T  L  E  S  G  A  Y
S  Q  U  A  B  B  L  E  S  P  K  V  A  W  T  H
```

Total number of marks	25
First time score	....
Score after revision	....

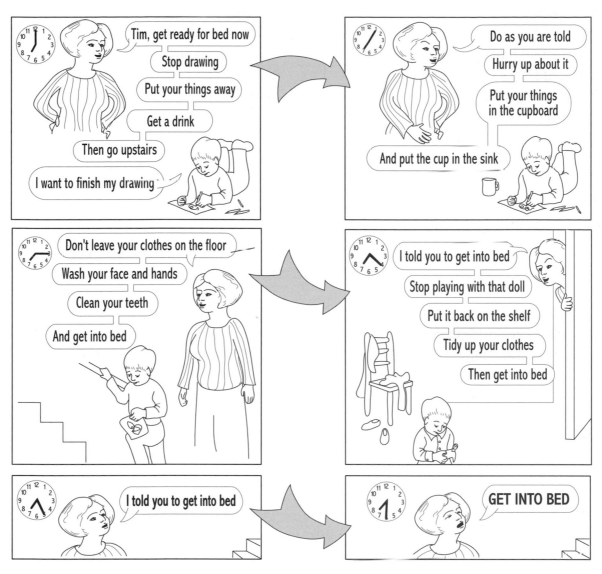

1 How many commands (orders) was Tim given at:

7.00?   ....

7.05?   ....

7.15?   ....

7.20?   ....

7.25?   ....

7.30?   ....

total commands in half an hour?   ....

2 How many commands were given using the word

i   'bed'?   ....

ii 'stop'?   ....

iii 'put'?   ....

3 What is the most likely reason that Tim did not do as he was asked?
   A he didn't hear his mother
   B he didn't like being shouted at
   C there were too many commands
   D he was deaf

4 Would these other actions by his mother be more successful in getting Tim to bed?

Yes/No

i   empty threats

ii   smacking

iii destroying his drawing

iv   negotiating

1   Commands given to Tim at

7.00	**5**
7.05	**4**
7.15	**4**
7.20	**5**
7.25	**1**
7.30	**1**
total	**20**

2   Commands – 'bed' **6**

                'stop' **2**

                'put' **4**

3   The most likely reason that Tim did not do as he was asked was that **there were too many commands**.

4   i   **No**. Empty threats do not work.

     ii   **No**. It is never necessary to correct a child by smacking, shaking or other forms of physical punishment. It might damage the child. It also teaches the child that it is alright to attack someone who is smaller than yourself.

     iii   **No**. This is likely to upset Tim and damage the relationship between him and his mother.

     iv   **Yes**. Negotiating a settlement between Tim and his mother means that Tim is much more likely to be cooperative. (See exercise 48)

Total number of marks	14
First time score	....
Score after revision	....

Sam's mother tried a different strategy to make for an easier bedtime.

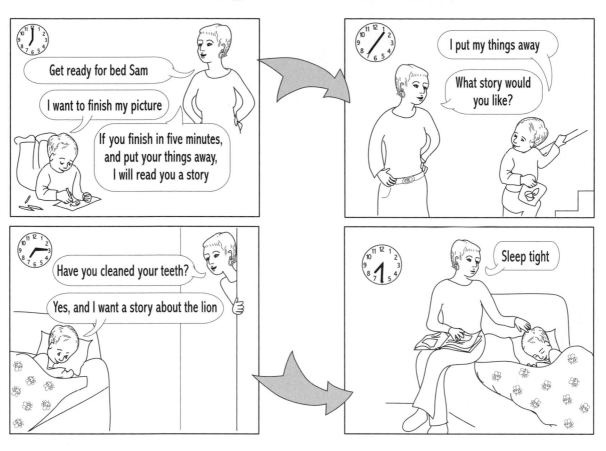

1 How many commands was Sam given?
A none
B 1
C 2
D 3

2 How many commands can most young children be expected to remember at any one time?
A 1–2
B 3–4
C 5–6
D 7–8

3 In picture 1 above, did Sam's mother
A give him orders
B let him dictate to her
C negotiate with him
D threaten him?

4 What is the most likely reason that Sam was co-operative?
A he would be punished if he disobeyed
B he knew he had to do as he was told
C there were too many commands
D he enjoys having stories read to him

| praising | not speaking | appearing to be uninterested | letting the child choose |
| looking away | cuddles | not touching the child | smiling |

5 Select four of the above actions that show approval of good behaviour:

i ....

ii ....

iii ....

iv ....

6 Select four of the above actions that show disapproval of naughty behaviour

i ....

ii ....

iii ....

iv ....

1 Sam's mother gave him only **1** command: 'Get ready for bed Sam'.

2 Most young children can retain only **1–2** commands at a time.

3 Sam's mother **negotiated with him**. Negotiation often works better than shouting or threatening in order to get children to co-operate.

4 The most likely reason that Sam was co-operative was that **he enjoys having stories read to him**.

5 Actions that show approval for good behaviour are (in any order):
praising
cuddles
smiling
letting the child choose

6 Actions that show disapproval of naughty behaviour (in any order):
looking away
not speaking
appearing to be uninterested
not touching the child

Total number of marks	12
First time score	....
Score after revision	....

True or false?   Yes/No

1   A pre-school group takes the place of home

2   A nursery school is one type of pre-school group

3   All children are ready for a pre-school group when they are 2 years old

4   Attendance at a pre-school group is compulsory

5   Play schools are for play and not education

6   Parent-and-toddler groups are only for toddlers (1 year to 2½ years)

7   Parent-and-toddler groups may take place in people's homes

8   Parents remain with their children at a parent-and-toddler group

9   All playgroup leaders and helpers must hold a relevant qualification

10   Playgroups must be registered with the Social Services Dept

11   Playgroups charge fees for the children attending them

12   Parents must stay with their children at playgroups

13   Nursery schools are for children aged 3–5 years

14   Nursery classes are for children aged 2–5 years

15   Most children at nursery schools attend for only half the day

16   Nursery schools provide the same kind of activities as playgroups

17   A nursery class is a class in an ordinary school

18   Each child should be encouraged to develop a positive self-image

19   Boys should be expected to behave in the same ways as girls

20   Boys and girls should be given the same opportunities

21   Gender stereotyping is treating boys and girls differently

22   When a child reaches 5 years of age, school is compulsory

1   **No**, but it provides additional opportunities.
2   **Yes**.
3   **No**. Many 2-year-olds are still too dependent on their parents and timid with others.
4   **No**.
5   **No**. Play is an essential part of their education because children learn as they play.
6   **No**. These groups are for any young children who are not yet ready to be separated from their parents.
7   **Yes**.
8   **Yes**.
9   **No,** but at least half should hold a relevant qualification.
10   **Yes**.
11   **Yes**.
12   **No**, but parents may be playgroup leaders or helpers.
13   **Yes**.
14   **No**. They give children aged 3–4 years the opportunity to begin school before the age of 5.
15   **Yes**.
16   **Yes**.
17   **Yes**.
18   **Yes**. Each should be treated as an individual with his/her own likes and dislikes.
19   **No**.
20   **Yes**.
21   **Yes**.
22   **Yes**.

Total number of marks	22
First time score	....
Score after revision	....

Josie enjoyed her first day at school. When the teacher asked her name she said that she was Josie Green and lived at 26 Manor Road. She came to school with a hanky and knew how to blow her nose. She was happy because she made some new friends and joined in all the activities.

When Josie wanted to go to the toilet, she was able to go on her own, and knew about washing her hands. She was able to use a knife and fork at dinner time. At the end of the school day, she put her coat on, did her shoes up, and ran off to greet her mum.

Josie's mum gave her a big hug and wanted to know all about her first day at school.

Linda did not enjoy her first day at school. She knew her name was Linda but when the teacher asked for Linda Brown she did not know that it meant her, and she did not know where she lived. She was unhappy because she felt lonely and didn't want to join in the activities.

Linda was not used to going to a strange toilet on her own, or washing her hands, or blowing her nose. At dinner time she was given a knife and fork, but at home she only used a spoon. At the end of the day she had to wait for someone to put her coat on and do her shoes up.

Linda's mum was late in meeting her and showed no interest in her first day at school.

1 Comparing Linda with Josie, list eight things that Linda did not know how to do.

i ....

ii ....

iii ....

iv ....

v ....

vi ....

vii ....

viii ....

2 On her first day at school,

i why was Josie happy? ....

....

ii why was Linda unhappy? ....

....

3 At the end of her first day,

i how did Josie's mum greet her? ....

....

ii How did Linda's mum behave? ....

....

1 When starting school, Linda did not know (in any order):
her full name
where she lived
how to blow her nose
how to go to the toilet on her own
how to wash her hands
how to use a knife and fork
how to put her coat on
how to do up her shoes

2 On her first day at school,
   i Josie was happy because **she made some new friends** and
                               joined in all the activities.
   ii Linda was unhappy because **she felt lonely** and
                              did not want to join in the activities.

3 i Josie's mum **gave her a big hug** and
                       wanted to know all about her first day at school.
   ii Linda's mum **was late in meeting her** and
                       showed no interest in her first day at school.

Total number of marks	16
First time score	....
Score after revision	....

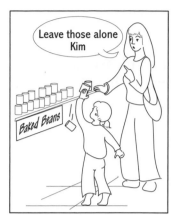
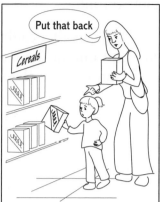
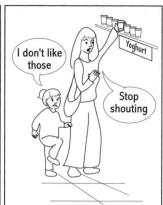
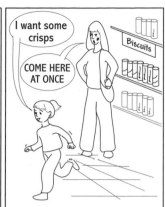
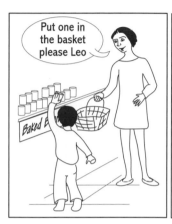
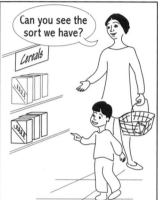
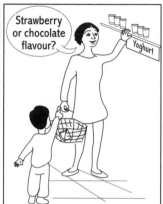
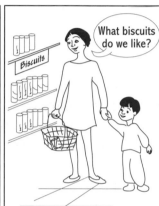

1 When the children were shopping with their mothers and reached the shelf:

	What did Kim's mother say?	**What did Leo's mother say?**
i with baked beans		
ii with cereals		
iii with yoghurts		
iv biscuits		

2 How many commands (orders) did Kim's mother give? ....

3 How many commands did Leo's mother give? ....

4 How many questions did Kim's mother ask which involved Kim in the shopping?......................

5 How many questions did Leo's mother ask which involved Leo in the shopping? ....

6 Which child was being encouraged in making choices – Kim or Leo? ....

7 Which child was ignored until he did something to annoy – Kim or Leo? ....

8 Who seemed to enjoy the visit to the shop more – Kim or Leo? ....

9 Who enjoyed shopping with their child more – Kim's mother or Leo's mother?..........................

1 When the children were shopping with their mothers and reached the shelf:

	Kim's mother said:	Leo's mother said:
i with baked beans	**Leave those alone Kim**	**Put one in the basket, please Leo**
ii with cereals	**Put that back**	**Can you see the sort we have?**
iii with yoghurts	**Stop shouting**	**Strawberry or chocolate flavour?**
iv biscuits	**Come here at once**	**What biscuits do we like?**

2 Kim was given **four** commands – 'Leave those alone'
                                      'Put that back'
                                      'Stop shouting'
                                      'Come here at once'

3 Leo was given **one** command – 'Put one in the basket'

4 **None**. No questions were asked of Kim.

5 Leo's mother asked him **three** questions – 'Can you see the sort we have?'
                                              'Would you like strawberry or chocolate flavour?'
                                              'What biscuits do we like?'

6 **Leo** was encouraged to make choices.

7 **Kim** was ignored until she did something to annoy.

8 **Leo** seemed to enjoy the visit to the shop more than Kim.

9 **Leo's mother** enjoyed shopping with her child more than Kim's mother.

Total number of marks   16
First time score   ....
Score after revision   ....

SECTION 6 FOOD

CONTENTS

1 Two of the nutrients in food are fats and
carbohydrates. Which are the other three?
 A fibre, minerals, vitamins
 B fibre, proteins, vitamins
 C proteins, minerals, vitamins
 D proteins, vitamins, water

2 Which of the following foods contains only
one nutrient?
 A meat
 B nuts
 C cheese
 D sugar

3 Carbohydrates include:
 A starch and fat
 B starch and sugar
 C sugar and fat
 D sugar, starch and fat

4 Which of the following provides the most
material for body growth and repair?
 A carbohydrates
 B fats
 C proteins
 D vitamins

5 Which foods all have a high protein content?
 A fish, eggs, beef
 B milk, cheese, cabbage
 C cheese, beans, butter
 D cream, bread, potatoes

6 Which of the following is not found in milk?
 A fat
 B starch
 C protein
 D sugar

7 Which vitamin is found in nearly all foods?
 A vitamin A
 B vitamin C
 C vitamin D
 D vitamin E

8 Which vitamins are often added to breakfast
cereals?
 A vitamins A and D
 B vitamins C and D
 C vitamins D and E
 D B vitamins

9 Which provide most of the body's energy?
 A vitamins and protein
 B protein and carbohydrates
 C carbohydrates and fats
 D fats and vitamins

10 Weight for weight, which of these foods has
the highest energy value?
 A apples
 B butter
 C milk
 D ice cream

11 Which of these foods contains the most
vitamin C?
 A bread
 B butter
 C cheese
 D tomatoes

12 Iron is required in the diet for:
 A making red blood cells
 B growth of nails
 C prevention of rickets
 D strengthening of teeth

13 In which of the following are both foods a
good source of iron?
 A cheese and beef
 B cheese and watercress
 C beef and milk
 D beef and liver

14 Calcium is required in the diet for:
 A making blood
 B growth of nails
 C prevention of anaemia
 D strengthening of bones

15 In which of the following are both foods a
good source of calcium?
 A white bread and cheese
 B cheese and tomatoes
 C bread and honey
 D meat and green vegetables

16 Fibre in the diet helps to prevent:
 A indigestion
 B constipation
 C coeliac disease
 D anaemia

1 Besides carbohydrates and fats, the other three nutrients in food are **proteins, minerals, vitamins**.

2 **Sugar** contains only one nutrient – it is 100% carbohydrate.

3 Carbohydrates include **starch and sugar.**

4 **Proteins** provide the most material for growth and repair of the body.

5 **Fish, eggs and beef** have a high protein content.

6 **Starch** is not found in milk.

7 **Vitamin E** is found in nearly all foods.

8 **B vitamins** are often added to breakfast cereals. The B group of vitamins contains a number of vitamins including thiamine (B_1), riboflavin (B_2), B_6, folic acid (folate) and niacin.

9 **Carbohydrates and fats** provide most of the body's energy.

10 Weight for weight **butter** has a higher energy value than apples, milk or ice cream because it has a very high fat content.

11 **Tomatoes** contain more vitamin C than bread, butter or cheese.

12 Iron is required in the diet for **making red blood cells**.

13 **Beef and liver** are good sources of iron.

14 Calcium is required in the diet to **strengthen bones**.

15 **White bread and cheese** are good sources of calcium. Calcium is added to white bread by government regulation.

16 Fibre in the diet helps prevent **constipation**.

Total number of marks	16
First time score	....
Score after revision	....

1 Additives are:
  A extra vitamins and minerals in food
  B extra nutrients added to food
  C substances added to food
  D synthetic (man-made) substances

2 Natural additives are:
  A salt, sugar, vinegar
  B tartrazine and sunset yellow
  C saccharin and sugar
  D vinegar and saccharin

3 Synthetic additives are:
  A carotene and vinegar
  B salt and tartrazine
  C saccharin and sugar
  D saccharin and sunset yellow

4 Preservatives are added to food to:
  A stop fatty foods from becoming rancid
  B protect it against microbes
  C prevent substances from separating
  D enable substances to mix together

5 The ingredients on food labels are listed in:
  A no particular order
  B alphabetical order
  C the amount present, starting with the largest
  D the amount present, starting with the least

6 E numbers are given to:
  A manufactured foods
  B all types of food
  C all ingredients in food
  D additives used in foods

7 Anti-oxidants are added to foods to:
  A stop fatty foods from becoming rancid
  B protect it against microbes
  C prevent substances from separating
  D enable substances to mix together

8 Emulsifiers are added to food to:
  A stop fatty foods from becoming rancid
  B protect it against microbes
  C prevent substances from separating
  D enable substances to mix together

9 Stabilisers are added to food to:
  A stop fatty foods from becoming rancid
  B protect it against microbes
  C prevent substances from separating
  D enable substances to mix together

10 Flavour enhancers
  A stop lumps forming in powdery foods
  B are used in low-calorie foods
  C are used to make food look attractive
  D stimulate the taste buds

11 Anti-caking agents
  A stop lumps forming in powdery foods
  B are used in low-calorie foods
  C are used to make food look attractive
  D stimulate the taste buds

12 Colourings
  A stop lumps forming in powdery foods
  B are used in low-calorie foods
  C are used to make food look attractive
  D stimulate the taste buds

13 Sweeteners
  A stop lumps forming in powdery foods
  B are used in low-calorie foods
  C are used to make food look attractive
  D stimulate the taste buds

14 Vitamins and minerals are often added to food to:
  A make the food look better
  B make the food taste better
  C replace those lost as the food is processed
  D increase the protein content

15 Some additives can:
  A increase the appetite
  B decrease the appetite
  C cause digestive problems in children
  D cause behaviour problems in children

16 Which additives have been linked with hyperactivity in children?
  A sugar and vinegar
  B tartrazine and sodium benzoate
  C saccharin and vitamins
  D sodium benzoate and salt

For more about additives see Topic 56

1 Additives are **substances added to food**. Some additives are natural (obtained from nature), others are synthetic (man-made).

2 Natural additives are **salt, sugar and vinegar**.

3. Synthetic additives are **saccharin and sunset yellow**.

4 Preservatives are added to food to **protect against microbes** spoiling the food.

5 The ingredients on food labels are listed in **the amount present, starting with the largest**.

6 E numbers are given to **additives used in foods**. Some come from plants and animals, others are synthetic (man-made).

7 Anti-oxidants are added to foods to **stop fatty foods from becoming rancid**.

8 Emulsifiers are added to foods to **enable substances to mix together** that would normally separate, for example oil and water.

9 Stabilisers are added to food to **prevent substances from separating**.

10 Flavour enhancers **stimulate the taste buds** and make food taste stronger, e.g. monosodium glutamate.

11 Anti-caking agents **stop lumps forming in powdery foods**.

12 Colourings **are used to make food look attractive**.

13 Sweeteners, for example saccharin, **are used in low-calorie foods**.

14 Vitamins and minerals, for example thiamine, riboflavin, folic acid and niacin, are often added to food to **replace those lost as the food is processed**.

15 Some additives can **cause behaviour problems in children**.

16 **Tartrazine and sodium benzoate** have been linked with hyperactivity in children, as have sunset yellow, carmoisine and ponceau.

Total number of marks	16
First time score	....
Score after revision	....

1 The word 'diet' means:
A eating a restricted range of foods
B the same as 'going on a diet'
C the same as 'dieting'
D the type of food that is usually eaten

2 'A balanced diet' contains:
A equal amounts of all the nutrients
B equal amounts of nutrients and fibre
C suitable amounts of nutrients
D suitable amounts of nutrients and fibre

3 People with diabetes need a diet
A containing no sugar
B containing no carbohydrates
C containing a regular amount of carbohydrates
D low in carbohydrates and fat

4 Children with coeliac disease need a gluten-free diet. This means they cannot eat:
A bread
B cornflakes
C rice
D potatoes

5 Deficiency diseases are:
A infectious
B contagious
C diet-related
D allergy-related

6 A shortage of iron in the diet results in:
A anaemia
B rickets
C scurvy
D night-blindness

7 Calcium in the diet is needed:
A to build strong muscles
B to make enough blood
C for strong bones and teeth
D for good eyesight

8 Which is not one of the B vitamins?
A thiamine
B folic acid
C riboflavin
D fluoride

9 A shortage of vitamin C in the diet leads to:
A anaemia
B rickets
C scurvy
D night-blindness

10 A shortage of vitamin D in the diet of children results in:
A anaemia
B rickets
C scurvy
D night-blindness

11 Which two vitamins are found mainly in fats?
A A and B
B A and C
C A and D
D B and C

12 Nourishing foods are those containing:
A fibre, proteins, vitamins
B fibre, vitamins, minerals
C proteins, fibre, flavour
D proteins, vitamins, minerals

13 Vegetarians do not eat:
A meat or dairy products
B meat or fish
C fish or eggs
D meat or eggs

14 Pulses (peas and beans) are especially useful in the diet of vegetarians because they supply:
A carbohydrates
B minerals
C vitamins
D protein

15 A vegan diet consists mainly of:
A cereals, milk, fruit, vegetables
B eggs, milk, fruit, vegetables
C cereals, fruit, vegetables, pulses
D fruit, vegetables, cereals, eggs

16 Vegans need to supplement their diet with:
A vitamin B_1
B vitamin B_2
C vitamin B_6
D vitamin B_{12}

1 The word 'diet' means **the type of food that is usually eaten**.

2 'A balanced diet' contains **suitable amounts of nutrients and fibre**.

3 People with diabetes need a diet **containing a regular amount of carbohydrates**.

4 Children with coeliac disease need a gluten-free diet and cannot eat **bread**. Also they cannot eat any foods containing wheat, barley, rye or oats.

5 Deficiency diseases are **diet-related** and occur when essential items in the diet are absent or in short supply.

6 A shortage of iron in the diet results in **anaemia**.

7 Calcium in the diet is needed **for strong bones and teeth**.

8 Thiamine, folic acid and riboflavin all belong to the B group of vitamins, **fluoride** does not.

9 A shortage of vitamin C in the diet results in **scurvy**.

10 A shortage of vitamin D in the diet of children results in **rickets**. Calcium and vitamin D are both essential to build strong bones.

11 Vitamins **A and D** are found mainly in fats.

12 Nourishing foods are those containing **proteins, vitamins and minerals**.

13 Vegetarians do not eat **meat or fish**.

14 Pulses (peas and beans) are especially useful in the diet of vegetarians because they supply **protein**.

15 A vegan diet consists mainly of **cereals, fruit, vegetables, pulses**.

16 Vegans need to supplement their diet with **vitamin B$_{12}$** because this vitamin occurs only in animal products.

Total number of marks	16
First time score	....
Score after revision	....

1 Weaning is:
- A the time when breast-/bottle-feeding ceases
- B the stage when babies become able to chew
- C the gradual introduction of solid foods
- D the gradual change from a milk diet to one based on a variety of foods.

2 The recommended time to begin weaning is at about:
- A 2 months old
- B 4 months old
- C 6 months old
- D 8 months old

3 Babies who are weaned too early may suffer from indigestion because young babies cannot:
- A digest starch
- B digest sugar
- C digest fat
- D digest protein

4 Babies who are weaned too early may:
- A refuse to eat weaning foods
- B develop food allergies
- C make their gums sore
- D lead to a feeding problem

5 When several months old, babies need foods containing:
- A fibre and sugar
- B sugar and starch
- C starch and fibre
- D starch and fat

6 From about the age of 6 months babies become able to:
- A swallow
- B chew
- C digest
- D taste

7 Drinking from a cup usually begins about the age of:
- A 4 months
- B 6 months
- C 8 months
- D 10 months

8 It is recommended that babies over 6 months old are given:
- A skimmed milk
- B semi-skimmed milk
- C infant formula
- D 'follow-on' milk

9 It is recommended that children over 1 year old be given cows' milk in the form of:
- A skimmed milk
- B semi-skimmed milk
- C whole milk
- D unpasteurised milk

10 Most babies have given up breast- or bottle-feeding at least during the day by:
- A 9 months old
- B 1 year old
- C 15 months old
- D 18 months old

11 When several months old, babies need foods containing more:
- A sugar
- B salt
- C iron
- D vitamin D

12 A weaning food containing iron is:
- A strawberry cheesecake puree
- B rice cakes
- C beef and vegetable puree
- D ice cream

13 Solid foods such as rusks and sandwiches
- A should never be given to babies
- B should always be mashed up first
- C can be given to babies who can chew
- D can be given to babies over 1 year old

14 Older babies who are thirsty should be given:
- A high-sugar fruit juice
- B low-calorie squash
- C weak tea
- D water

1 Weaning is the **gradual change from a milk diet to one based on a variety of foods**.

2 The recommended time to begin weaning is when the baby is **6 months old**.

3 Babies who are weaned too early may suffer from indigestion because the digestive system has not yet developed enough to **digest starch**.

4 Babies who are weaned too early may **develop food allergies**.

5 When several months old babies need foods containing **starch and fibre**.

6 From about the age of 6 months babies become able to **chew**.

7 Drinking from a cup usually begins about the age of **6 months**.

8 It is recommended that babies over 6 months old are given '**follow-on**' **milk**.

9 It is recommended that children over 1 year old be given cow's milk in the form of **whole milk**.

10 Most babies have given up breast- or bottle-feeding at least during the daytime by **9 months old**.

11 When several months old babies need food containing more **iron**.

12 A weaning food containing iron is **beef and vegetable puree**. Meat and vegetables both contain iron.

13 Solid foods such as rusks and sandwiches **can be given to babies who can chew**.

14 Older babies who are thirsty should be given **water**.

Total number of marks	14
First time score	....
Score after revision	....

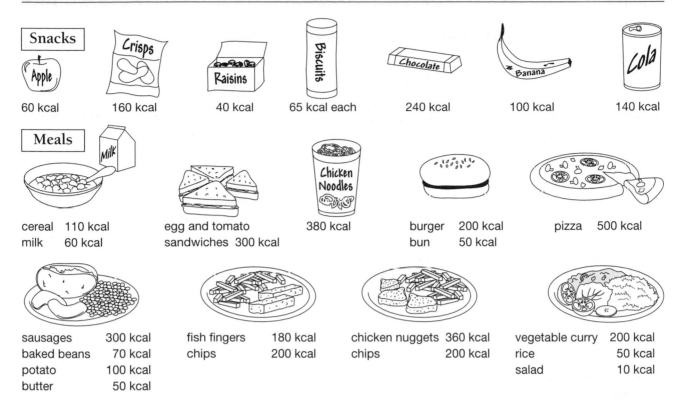

Snacks

Apple 60 kcal

Crisps 160 kcal

Raisins 40 kcal

Biscuits 65 kcal each

Chocolate 240 kcal

Banana 100 kcal

Cola 140 kcal

Meals

Milk

cereal 110 kcal
milk 60 kcal

egg and tomato
sandwiches 300 kcal

Chicken Noodles 380 kcal

burger 200 kcal
bun 50 kcal

pizza 500 kcal

sausages 300 kcal
baked beans 70 kcal
potato 100 kcal
butter 50 kcal

fish fingers 180 kcal
chips 200 kcal

chicken nuggets 360 kcal
chips 200 kcal

vegetable curry 200 kcal
rice 50 kcal
salad 10 kcal

Energy intake of three 6-year-old children for one day
Note: kcal = kilocalorie; kilocalories are commonly referred to as calories.

	Child X	kcal	Child Y	kcal	Child Z	kcal
Breakfast	cereal and milk bun with butter	....	banana milk	....	cereal and milk chicken noodles	....
Midday	chicken nuggets chips baked beans	....	vegetable curry rice salad	....	sausages baked beans potato and butter	....
Tea-time and snacks	2 burgers and buns banana apple 4 biscuits	....	sandwiches raisins apple 1 biscuit	....	pizza chocolate bar 2 cans of cola 2 pkts crisps	....
Total kcal						
Kilojoules						

1 Complete the table above:
   i   calculate how much energy in kilocalories (kcal) each child consumed during the day.
   ii convert the totals from kilocalories (kcal) to kilojoules (kJ). 1 kcal = 4.184 kJ.

2 Which midday meal contains the most energy?..

3 Which snack without fat contains the most energy?...

4 Which child, X, Y or Z:

   i   may be a vegetarian? ....   ii ate no fruit or vegetables? ....

   iii was most likely to be overweight? ....   iv was most likely to be underweight? ....

1   Energy intake of three 6-year-old children for one day

	Child X	kcal	Child Y	kcal	Child Z	kcal
Breakfast	cereal and milk bun with butter	170 100	banana milk	100 60	cereal and milk chicken noodles	170 380
Midday	chicken nuggets chips baked beans	360 200 70	vegetable curry rice salad	200 50 10	sausages baked beans potato and butter	300 70 150
Tea-time and snacks	2 burgers and buns banana apple 4 biscuits	500 100 60 260	sandwiches raisins apple 1 biscuit	300 40 60 65	pizza chocolate bar 2 cans of cola 2 pkts crisps	500 240 280 320
Total kcal.....		1820		885		2410
Kilojoules		7615		3703		10,083

2 Chicken nuggets, baked beans and chips contained the most energy (630 kcal).

3 Cola contained 140 kcal of energy even though it lacked fat.

4 i **Child Y** may have been vegetarian.

ii **Child Z** ate no fruit or vegetables.

iii **Child X** was closest to the average daily energy intake of 7.25 MJ.

iv **Child Z** was most likely to be overweight, especially if this day's intake was typical and the child took little exercise.

v **Child Y** was most likely to be underweight if this day's intake was typical.

Total number of marks   40
First time score   ....
Score after revision   ....

Michael and Christopher are five-year-old identical twins. They are healthy boys and full of life. But they are also impulsive, have problems concentrating, cannot stay still, and tend to throw temper tantrums. This makes them difficult to manage both at home and at school.

Their mother accepted an invitation to take part in an experiment to see if additives in the twins' diet were affecting their behaviour. Before the experiment, the twins were given tests to measure their concentration and IQ, and they achieved identical scores. Then Michael was put on an additive-free diet.

After two weeks the twins' mother was amazed by the improvement in Michael's behaviour. He was calmer, less fidgety, and out-performed his brother in the concentration and IQ tests.

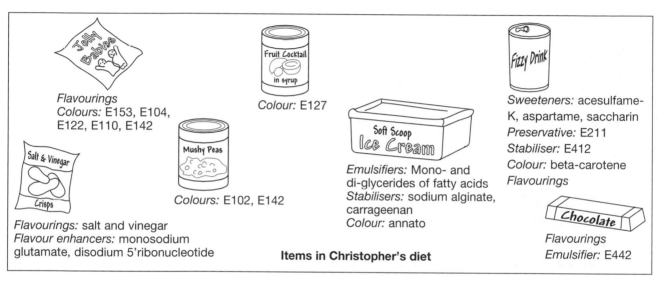

Flavourings
Colours: E153, E104, E122, E110, E142

Colour: E127

Emulsifiers: Mono- and di-glycerides of fatty acids
Stabilisers: sodium alginate, carrageenan
Colour: annato

Sweeteners: acesulfame-K, aspartame, saccharin
Preservative: E211
Stabiliser: E412
Colour: beta-carotene
Flavourings

Colours: E102, E142

Flavourings: salt and vinegar
Flavour enhancers: monosodium glutamate, disodium 5'ribonucleotide

Flavourings
Emulsifier: E442

Items in Christopher's diet

Source: Based on an experiment by Professor Jim Stevenson of the University of Southampton

1   Match the items in Michael's new diet below with those in Christopher's diet shown above.

Michael's new diet:	**Christopher's diet:**
ready salted crisps	....
home-made lemonade	....
fresh vegetables	....
fresh fruit	....
additive-free yoghurt	....
dried banana chips	....
peanuts	....

2   Name the different types of additive in Christopher's diet (those words in italics):

....

....

3   Which food has the most types of (i) colours? ....

(ii) additives? ....

4   How did the additive-free diet affect Michael?...

....

1 Matching the items in Michael's new diet below with those in Christopher's diet:

Michael's new diet:	Christopher's diet:
ready salted crisps	**salt and vinegar crisps**
home-made lemonade	**fizzy drink**
fresh vegetables	**mushy peas**
fresh fruit	**tinned fruit cocktail in syrup**
additive-free yoghurt	**ice cream**
dried banana chips	**jelly babies** (alternative answer – chocolate)
peanuts	**chocolate** (alternative answer – jelly babies)

2 The types of additive in Christopher's diet were:
flavourings
flavour enhancers
colours
emulsifiers
stabilisers
sweeteners
preservatives

3 (i) The **jelly babies** contained the most colours.
(ii) The **fizzy drink** contained the most additives.

4 After two weeks on an additive-free diet Michael was **calmer, less fidgety, and out-performed his brother in the IQ and concentration tests.** (1 mark)

Total number of marks   17
First time score   ....
Score after revision   ....

1 Food hygiene is concerned with the:
A care of food
B preparation of food
C storage of food
D care, preparation and storage of food

2 The four golden rules of food hygiene are:

i   keep food c __ __ __ n

ii keep fresh food c __ __ __

iii cook food t __ __ __ __ __ __ __ ly

iv do not eat food past its __ __ __   __ __ date

3 Bacteria thrive best in food which is:
A warm, moist and contains starch
B warm, moist and contains fat
C warm, moist and contains sugar
D warm, moist and contains protein

4 In the right conditions for growth, bacteria can multiply (double) every:
A 10 minutes
B 20 minutes
C 30 minutes
D 40 minutes

5 It is recommended that refrigerators are kept at a temperature between:
A 0°C and 2°C
B 0°C and 4°C
C 1°C and 3°C
D 1°C and 5°C

6 The low temperature in a refrigerator
A kills bacteria
B stops their growth
C slows down their growth
D does not affect their growth

7 The temperature of −18°C in a freezer
A kills bacteria
B stops their growth
C slows down their growth
D does not affect their growth

8 Food containing food-poisoning bacteria
A does not look fit to eat
B does not taste fit to eat
C does not smell fit to eat
D may look, taste and smell fit to eat

Food-poisoning cases in the UK

No. of cases (to the nearest thousand)

27 000 — 1986
56 000 — 1989
68 000 — 1992
93 000 — 1995
105 000 — 1998
95 000 — 2001

9 From the bar chart above,

i   by which year had the number of cases of food poisoning doubled since 1986? ....

ii how many years after 1986 did it take for the cases to double? ....

iii by which year had the number of cases almost quadrupled since 1986? ....

10 The rise in the number of food-poisoning cases is most likely due to:
A a similar increase in the population
B inadequate hygiene
C changing eating patterns
D a greater use of additives

11 To prevent food poisoning, rats and mice should be kept away from the kitchen because:
A they give off a nasty smell
B some people are frightened of them
C their droppings contain bacteria
D food which they nibble does not look nice

12 Which of these causes of food poisoning
   Salmonella   Staphylococcus
   Clostridium   Campylobacter   E. coli

i   are found in the nose, throat and pus?

   ....

ii have spores which can withstand boiling?

   ....

iii is the most common cause?

   ....

1 Food hygiene is concerned with the **care, preparation and storage of food**.

2 The four golden rules of food hygiene are:
   i   keep food **clean**
   ii keep fresh food **cold** when being stored
   iii cook food **thoroughly**
   iv do not eat food past its **use by** date

3 Food-poisoning bacteria thrive best in food which is **warm, moist and contains protein**, for example cooked and uncooked meat and poultry, gravy, egg dishes and milk.

4 In the right conditions for growth, bacteria in food can multiply every **20 minutes**.

5 It is recommended that refrigerators are kept at a temperature between **1°C and 5°C**.

6 The low temperature in a refrigerator **slows down the growth of bacteria**.

7 The temperature of minus 18°C in a freezer **stops bacterial growth**.

8 Food containing harmful bacteria **may look, taste and smell fit to eat**.

9 i   The number of cases of food poisoning had doubled by **1989**.
   ii The number of cases had doubled in **3** years.
   iii The number of cases had almost quadrupled by **1998**.

10 The rise in the number of food-poisoning cases is most likely due to **inadequate hygiene**.

11 To prevent food poisoning, rats and mice should be kept away from the kitchen because **of bacteria in their droppings**.

12 i   **Staphylococcus** bacteria are found in the nose, throat and pus.
   ii The spores of **Clostridium** can withstand boiling for prolonged periods.
   iii **Campylobacter** is the most common cause of food poisoning.
       Note: **Salmonella** and **E. coli** bacteria usually live harmlessly in the intestines of humans and animals. They cause food-poisoning when food is contaminated by excreta (faeces) of humans or animals.

Total number of marks	19
First time score	....
Score after revision	....

Across

1 The name for tooth decay (6)

3 A baby who is cutting a tooth might have a __ __ __ patch on the cheek (3)

6 The first teeth usually appear in this part of the jaw (5)

7 Children need to be taught to __ __ __ __ __ their teeth (5)

9 The first tooth to come through is usually this type (7)

11 When a tooth does this it can be painful (6)

12 This type of tooth only appears when the permanent set come through (5)

15 Some teeth come through __ __ __ __ __ly, others are much slower (5)

17 Produced when bacteria in the mouth come into contact with sugar (4)

18 Continuously forms on the teeth (6)

19 Flu __ __ __ __ e helps to prevent tooth decay (4)

Down

1 A mineral which strengthens teeth (7)

2 A pain in this part of the head is not a symptom of teething (3)

4 A person who is skilled at preventing and treating problems with teeth (7)

5 Milk teeth start to f __ __ __ out from the age of five (3)

8 Sticky f __ __ __ adheres to the teeth and encourages tooth decay (3)

10 __ __ __ __ __ __ __ visits to the dentist help to prevent tooth problems (7)

13 If bronchitis, fever, or convulsions __ __ __ __ __ at the time when teeth are coming through they will not be due to teething (5)

14 Vitamins, A, C __ __ __ D help to build strong, healthy teeth (3)

16 When their milk teeth fall out, some children like to __ __ __ __ them for the 'tooth fairy' (4)

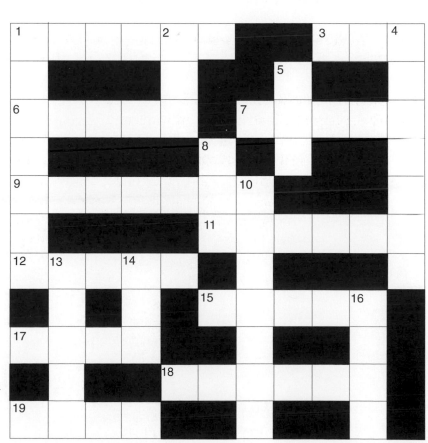

1 C	A	R	I	2 E	S			3 R	E	4 D
A				A			5 A			E
6 L	O	W	E	R		7 C	L	E	A	N
C				8 O		L				T
9 I	N	C	I	S	O	10 R				I
U				11 D	E	C	A	Y	S	
12 M	13 O	L	14 A	R		G				T
	C		N		15 Q	U	I	C	16 K	
17 A	C	I	D			L			E	
	U			18 P	L	A	Q	U	E	
19 O	R	I	D			R			P	

Total number of marks   20
First time score   ....
Score after revision   ....

SECTION 7 HEALTH AND SAFETY

CONTENTS

CONTENTS

1 Pathogens are commonly called:
  A microbes
  B bacteria
  C viruses
  D germs

2 Bacteria multiply by:
  A producing spores
  B dividing into two
  C dividing into many parts
  D producing particles

3 Viruses can only grow and multiply:
  A in living cells
  B in water
  C in dead cells
  D in soil

4 Contagious diseases are spread by:
  A contact with an infectious person
  B droplet infection
  C antibodies
  D spores

5 Incubation of a disease is:
  A the ability of a body to resist infection
  B a change in the body which indicates disease
  C the time between entry of germs and appearance of symptoms
  D the time during which germs can be spread

6 Immunity is:
  A the ability of the body to resist infection
  B a change in the body which indicates diease
  C the time between entry of germs and appearance of symptoms
  D the time during which germs can be spread

7 The infectious stage is the time:
  A when germs enter the body
  B during which symptoms appear
  C between entry of germs and appearance of symptoms
  D during which germs can be spread

Notification of infectious diseases		
	1990	**2000**
Tuberculosis	5010	5915
Whooping cough	14125	658
Scarlet fever	6988	1879
Meningitis	2369	2251
Measles	12703	2265
Mumps	4058	2111
Rubella	11070	1587

Source: PHLS Communicable Disease Surveillance

8 List the diseases given in the table from most common to least common in 1990:

....

....

....

....

....

....

....

9 Comparing 1990 with 2000, which disease had shown the:

i   greatest fall in numbers?

....

ii   second greatest fall in numbers?

....

iii   the lowest fall in numbers?

....

iv   an increase in numbers?

....

1 Pathogens (microbes that cause disease) are commonly called **germs**.

2 Bacteria multiply by **dividing into two**.

3. Viruses can only grow and multiply when they are **in living cells**.

4 Contagious diseases are spread by **contact with an infectious person**. They can also be spread by contact with objects that have been in contact with an infectious person.

5 Incubation of a disease is **the time between entry of germs and appearance of symptoms**.

6 Immunity is **the ability of the body to resist infection**.

7 The infectious stage is the time **during which germs can be spread**.

8 **Whooping cough**
Measles
Rubella
Scarlet fever
Tuberculosis
Mumps
Meningitis

9 i   **Whooping cough** showed the greatest fall in numbers (13467).
   ii   **Measles** showed the second greatest fall in numbers (10438).
   ii   **Meningitis** showed the least drop in numbers (118).
   iii **Tuberculosis** showed an increase in numbers (905).

Total number of marks	18
First time score	....
Score after revision	....

Chicken pox	Rubella	Tuberculosis	Polio (Poliomyelitis)
Scarlet fever	Measles	Whooping cough (Pertussis)	Diphtheria
Meningitis	Hib (*Haemophilus influenzae* type B)	Mumps	Tetanus

1 Name the infectious disease above characterised by:

i   small red spots which turn into blisters then scabs ....

ii   painful swelling on one or both sides near the jaw...

iii long bouts of coughing which may end with a 'whoop'...

iv   a white layer forming on the throat...

v   muscles in the neck tighten and lock the jaw...

vi   cough with phlegm containing blood...

vii a red rash which appears on the face and spreads downwards..

2 Name the disease above which:

i   is dangerous in early pregnancy ....

ii   causes a range of illnesses including meningitis ....

iii may result in shingles...

iv   may cause sterility when it occurs in males over the age of 11..

v   can be caught from germs in the soil...

vi   causes inflammation of the lining (meninges) of the brain ....

3 The MMR vaccine protects against:

i ....   ii ....

iii ....

4 Name the five diseases that the 'five in one' vaccine protects against:

i   D __ __ __ __ __ __ __ __ __

ii   T __ __ __ __ __ __

iii P __ __ __ __

iv   H __ __

v   W __ __ __ __ __ __ __   __ __ __ __ __

5 The BCG vaccine protects against:...

1　i　small red spots which turn into blisters then scabs – **chicken pox**

　　ii　painful swelling on one or both sides near the jaw – **mumps**

　　iii　long bouts of coughing which may end in a 'whoop' – **whooping cough**

　　iv　a white layer forming on the throat – **diphtheria**

　　v　muscles in the neck tighten and lock the jaw – **tetanus**

　　vi　cough with phlegm containing blood – **tuberculosis**

　　vii　a red rash which appears on the face and spreads downwards – **measles**.

2　i　**Rubella** is dangerous to the unborn baby if the mother catches this disease in early pregnancy.

　　ii　**Hib** (*Haemophilus influenzae* type B) may cause meningitis.

　　iii　The **chicken pox** virus may remain in the body and cause shingles in later life.

　　iv　**Mumps** may cause sterility in males over the age of 11.

　　v　**Tetanus** can be caught from germs in the soil.

　　vi　**Meningitis** causes inflammation of the lining (meninges) of the brain.

3　The MMR vaccine protects against **measles**, **mumps** and **rubella**.

4　The 'five in one' vaccine protects against **diphtheria**, **tetanus**, **polio**, **Hib** and **whooping cough** (pertussis).

5　The BCG (*bacille Calmette-Guérin*) vaccine protects against **tuberculosis**.

Total number of marks	21
First time score	……..
Score after revision	……..

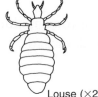

Louse (×20)

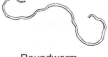

Roundworm (half size)

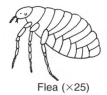

Flea (×25)

Itch mite (×20)

Threadworm (×2)

1 Which of these five parasites

i causes scabies? ....

ii can cause serious disease? ....

iii lives in clothing? ....

iv lives amongst hairs? ....

v lives in the skin? ....

vi lives in the human intestine? ....

vii lives in a dog's or cat's intestines? ....

2 Threadworms:
A burrow into the skin
B crawl amongst hairs
C move by jumping
D move by wriggling

3 Itch mites:
A burrow into the skin
B crawl amongst hairs
C move by jumping
D move by wriggling

4 Fleas:
A burrow into the skin
B crawl amongst hairs
C move by jumping
D move by wriggling

5 Lice:
A burrow into the skin
B crawl amongst hairs
C move by jumping
D move by wriggling

6 Roundworms lay eggs:
A in clothing
B in the skin
C around the anus
D in the intestine

7 Fleas lay eggs:
A in clothing
B in the skin
C around the anus
D in the intestine

8 Itch mites lay eggs:
A in clothing
B in the skin
C around the anus
D in the intestine

9 Threadworms lay eggs:
A in clothing
B in the skin
C around the anus
D in the intestine

10 Lice can be removed by:
A cleanliness
B wet combing
C applying lotion
D a special medicine

11 Threadworms can be removed by:
A cleanliness
B special shampoo
C applying lotion
D special medicine

12 Fleas can be removed by:
A cleanliness
B special shampoo
C applying lotion
D special medicine

13 Itch mites can be removed by:
A cleanliness
B special shampoo
C applying lotion
D special medicine

14
i Name this egg: ....
ii Which parasite was it laid by?

....

15 Name the parasites above that cause infection when their eggs are eaten:

i ....

ii ....

1 i **Itch mites** cause scabies.
ii **Roundworms** can cause serious disease (toxocariasis). Symptoms include fever, vomiting, pain in muscles and joints, and eyesight may be damaged.
iii **Fleas** live in clothing next to the skin.
iv The **louse** (plural: lice) lives amongst hairs.
v **Itch mites** live in the skin.
vi **Threadworms** live in the human intestine.
vii **Roundworms** live in dogs' and cats' intestines.

2 Threadworms **move by wriggling**.

3 Itch mites **burrow into the skin**.

4 Fleas **move by jumping**.

5 Lice **crawl amongst hairs**.

6 Roundworms lay eggs **in the intestine**.

7 Fleas lay eggs **in clothing**.

8 Itch mites lay eggs **in the skin**.

9 Threadworms lay eggs **around the anus**.

10 Lice can be removed by **wet combing**. After washing the hair using an ordinary shampoo, apply lots of conditioner to make it slippery, then comb with a fine-tooth comb to remove the lice.

11 Threadworms can be removed by **a special medicine**.

12 Fleas can be removed by **cleanliness**. They do not live long on clean people or on clothes and bedding which are regularly washed.

13 Itch mites can be removed by **applying lotion** to all parts of the skin from the neck to the soles of the feet.

14 i The egg is called a **nit**.
ii It was laid by a **louse** and glued to a hair.

15 **Threadworms** and **roundworms** infect the body when their eggs are eaten.

Total number of marks	23
First time score	....
Score after revision	....

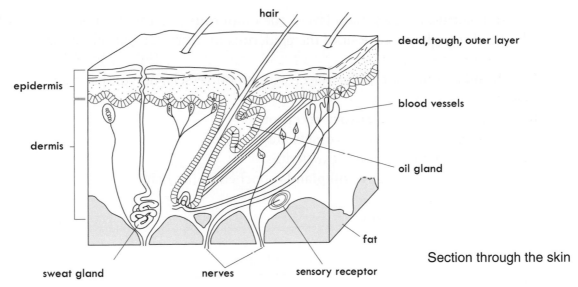

Section through the skin

1 Use the diagram above to fill in the missing words.

i   The skin consists of two main layers, the _ _ _ _ _ _ _ _ _ _ and the

   _ _ _ _ _ _ .

ii The _ _ _ _ , _ _ _ _ _ , outer layer of the epidermis protects the delicate
   tissues underneath.

iii The _ _ _ _ _ _ is the softer, inner layer with blood vessels, nerves, hairs and
   _ _ _ _ _ glands.

iv Pain is detected by the _ _ _ _ _ _ _ _ _ _ _ _ _ _ _ .

v   The skin bleeds when blood _ _ _ _ _ _ _ are damaged.

vi _ _ _ is stored in a layer under the skin.

vii Greasy skin is due to active _ _ _ _ _ _ _ s attached to the hairs.

2 Which vitamin can be made in the skin?
  A vitamin A
  B vitamin B
  C vitamin C
  D vitamin D

3 Ringworm is a skin complaint caused by:
  A bacteria
  B a fungus
  C a virus
  D tiny worms

4 Impetigo is a skin complaint caused by:
  A bacteria
  B a fungus
  C a virus
  D an allergy

5 Urticaria is the medical name for:
  A eczema
  B impetigo
  C plantar warts
  D nettle rash

6 Eating strawberries or shellfish may cause:
  A eczema
  B impetigo
  C plantar warts
  D nettle rash (hives)

7 Athlete's foot has the same cause as:
  A impetigo
  B ringworm
  C warts
  D eczema

8 Warts are caused by:
  A bacteria
  B a fungus
  C a virus
  D an allergy

9 Plantar warts occur on the:
  A hands
  B face
  C fingers
  D feet

1 i   The skin consists of two main layers, the **epidermis** and the **dermis**.   (2 marks)

    ii   The **dead**, **tough**, outer layer of the epidermis protects the delicate tissues underneath.   (1 mark)

   iii   The **dermis** is the softer, inner layer with blood vessels, nerves, hairs and **sweat** glands.   (2 marks)

   iv   Pain is detected by the **sensory receptors.**   (1 mark)

    v   The skin bleeds when blood **vessels** are damaged.   (1 mark)

   vi   **Fat** is stored in a layer under the dermis.   (1 mark)

  vii   Greasy skin is due to active **oil gland**s attached to the hairs.   (1 mark)

2   **Vitamin D** is made in the skin.

3   Ringworm is a skin complaint caused by **a fungus**.

4   Impetigo is a skin complaint caused by **bacteria**.

5   Urticaria is the medical name for **nettle rash**.

6   Eating strawberries or shellfish may cause **nettle rash (hives)** in people who are allergic to these foods.

7   Athlete's foot is **ringworm** of the feet.

8   Warts are caused by **a virus**.

9   Plantar warts occur on the soles of the **feet**. A plantar wart is also called a verruca.

Total number of marks	17
First time score	....
Score after revision	....

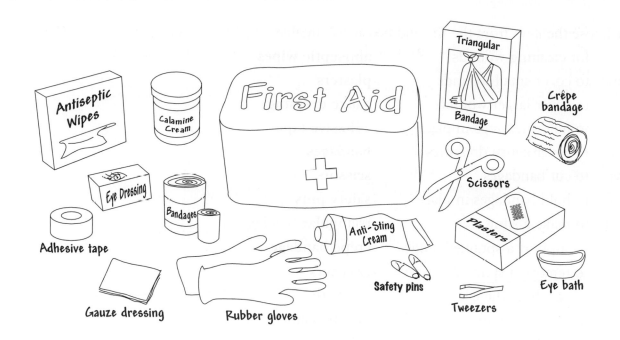

1 Choose the most suitable item from the first aid box (hint: the number of dashes in each label equals the number of letters in the answer):

i   for cleaning wounds   _ _ _ _ _ _ _ _ _ _   _ _ _ _ _

ii   to cover small wounds   _ _ _ _ _ _ _ _

iii   to cover larger wounds   _ _ _ _ _   _ _ _ _ _ _ _ _

iv   to hold dressings in place   _ _ _ _ _ _ _ _ _   _ _ _ _

v   to cover gauze dressings   _ _ _ _ _ _ _ _ _

vi   to cut bandages   _ _ _ _ _ _ _ _

vii   to hold bandages in place   _ _ _ _ _ _ _   _ _ _ _ _

viii to make a sling   _ _ _ _ _ _ _ _ _ _   _ _ _ _ _ _ _

ix   to support a sprained ankle   _ _ _ _ _   _ _ _ _ _ _ _

x   to remove a splinter   _ _ _ _ _ _ _ _

xi   for washing the eye   _ _ _   _ _ _ _

xii   to cover an injured eye   _ _ _   _ _ _ _ _ _ _

xiii for sunburn or chapped skin   _ _ _ _ _ _ _ _   _ _ _ _ _

xiv   for insect bites   _ _ _ _ - _ _ _ _ _   _ _ _ _ _

xv   when dealing with blood   _ _ _ _ _ _   _ _ _ _ _ _

1   Choose the item from the first aid box most suitable:

i	for cleaning wounds	**antiseptic wipes**
ii	to cover small wounds	**plasters**
iii	to cover larger wounds	**gauze dressing**
iv	to hold dressings in place	**adhesive tape**
v	to cover gauze dressings	**bandages**
vi	to cut bandages	**scissors**
vii	to hold bandages in place	**safety pins**
viii	to make a sling	**triangular bandage**
ix	to support a sprained ankle	**crêpe bandage**
x	to remove a splinter	**tweezers**
xi	for washing the eye	**eye bath**
xii	to cover an injured eye	**eye dressing**
xiii	for sunburn or chapped skin	**calamine cream**
xiv	for insect bites	**anti-sting cream**
xv	when dealing with blood	**rubber gloves**

Total number of marks   15
First time score   ....
Score after revision   ....

1 The first thing to do for a small cut or graze is:
   A cover with a plaster
   B apply antiseptic cream
   C wash and dry it with a clean towel
   D apply a bandage

2 The first thing to do for a wound with severe bleeding is to:
   A cover with a plaster
   B apply a bandage
   C apply antiseptic cream
   D apply pressure to the wound or nearest artery

3 A wounded person may be advised to have an injection against:
   A toxoplasmosis
   B tuberculosis
   C typhoid
   D tetanus

4 A bruise is caused by:
   A damage to the skin
   B damage to muscle tissue
   C bleeding under the skin
   D inflammation of a bone

5 To prevent a bruise from developing:
   A apply a cold compress
   B apply a hot compress
   C apply pressure to the area
   D apply calamine cream

6 For a nose bleed, ask the patient to:
   A put the head between the knees
   B lie down and pinch the nose
   C sit leaning backwards and pinch the nose
   D sit leaning forwards and pinch the nose

7 If you see someone receiving an electric shock, the first thing to do is to:
   A grasp his legs and pull him away
   B push him away with a metal object
   C use something damp to pull him away
   D switch off the current

8 A greenstick fracture is:
   A a bone which is bent
   B a broken bone
   C a bone cracked on one side
   D a chip off a bone

9 Something in the eye is best removed by:
   A using a handkerchief
   B washing it out
   C rubbing the eye
   D using tweezers

10 Immediate treatment for a small burn or scald is to:
   A rub in ointment
   B cover with oil
   C rub in butter
   D hold it under cold running water

11 Sunburn occurs more quickly at the seaside because:
   A the sun's rays are extra strong
   B sea breezes cool the skin
   C the air is less polluted
   D there is more ozone in the air

12 Excessive exposure to the sun can cause:
   A dry skin
   B oily skin
   C skin allergy
   D skin cancer

13 Cough mixture, tranquillisers, sleeping pills and contraceptive pills are all:
   A sedatives for children
   B causes of diarrhoea in children
   C causes of vomiting in children
   D common causes of poisoning in children

14 If a child swallows poison what do you **not** do?
   A keep calm
   B make the child sick
   C telephone a doctor or take to hospital
   D identify the poison to tell the doctor

1 The first thing to do for a small cut or graze is to **wash and dry it with a clean towel**. Bleeding from a small wound soon stops of its own accord and the scab which forms prevents infection. A plaster can be used if the wound keeps opening up.

2 For a wound with severe bleeding **apply pressure to the wound or nearest artery** to stop the bleeding.

3 A wounded person may be advised to have an injection against **tetanus**.

4 A bruise is caused by **bleeding under the skin**.

5 To prevent a bruise from developing **apply pressure to the area**.

6 For a nose bleed, ask the patient to **sit leaning forwards and pinch the nose**.

7 When a person is receiving an electric shock the first thing to do is to **switch off the current**. Avoid using anything metallic or damp, or allowing your hands to touch the casualty's flesh.

8 A greenstick fracture is **a bone cracked on one side**.

9 Something in the eye is best removed by **washing it out**.

10 Immediate treatment for a small burn or scald is to **hold it under cold running water** for 10 minutes, or put it into a water bath containing ice cubes. This removes the heat and stops the burning.

11 Sunburn occurs more quickly at the seaside because the **sun's rays are extra strong**. The skin receives rays directly from the sun and also from the sun's rays reflected off the water.

12 Excessive exposure to the sun can cause **skin cancer**.

13 Cough mixture, tranquillisers, sleeping pills and sedatives are all **common causes of poisoning in children**.

14 If a child swallows poison do *not* **make the child sick**, but keep calm, telephone a doctor or take the child to hospital, and identify the poison to tell the doctor.

| Total number of marks | 14 |
| Total number of marks   14 |
| First time score   .... |
| Score after revision   .... |

1 Match each of the brief descriptions below with one of the 12 common illnesses in the list.

being sick

red eyes and yellowish discharge

jerking movements of arms and legs

enlarged tissue behind the nose

difficulty in breathing

fungal infection of the mouth

yellowish discharge from the eye

a harsh cough in children under 4 years

infrequent passing of hard, dry stools

sensitivity to a particular substance

frequent passing of loose, watery stools

higher body temperature than normal

i   Swollen adenoids...

ii   Allergy   ....

iii   Asthma   ....

iv   Conjunctivitis   ....

v   Constipation   ....

vi   Convulsion   ....

vii   Croup   ....

viii   Diarrhoea   ....

xi   Fever   ....

x   Sticky eye   ....

xi   Thrush   ....

xii   Vomiting   ....

2 An acute illness is:
A short term
B long term
C mild
D severe

3 A chronic illness is:
A short term
B long term
C mild
D severe

4 Following a convulsion, the child needs to be placed in the recovery position, which is:
A lying on the back
B lying on the side
C lying on the front
D in a sitting position

5 The tonsils normally enlarge after the age of:
A 5 years and shrink after the age of 10
B 2 years and shrink after the age of 5
C 2 years and shrink after the age of 10
D 5 years and shrink after the age of 15

6 Children with diarrhoea are liable to become:
A hydrated
B rehydrated
C dehydrated
D bloated

7 A child with a fever should be:
A kept in warm room
B wrapped in a blanket
C given a warm bath
D allowed to cool off

1
i	Swollen adenoids	**enlarged tissue behind the nose**
ii	Allergy	**sensitivity to a particular substance**
iii	Asthma	**difficulty in breathing**
iv	Conjunctivitis	**red eyes often with a yellowish discharge**
v	Constipation	**infrequent passing of hard, dry stools**
vi	Convulsion	**jerking movements of arms and legs**
vii	Croup	**a harsh cough in children under 4 years**
viii	Diarrhoea	**frequent passing of loose, watery stools**
ix	Fever	**higher body temperature than normal**
x	Sticky eye	**yellowish discharge from the eye**
xi	Thrush	**fungal infection of the mouth**
xii	Vomiting	**being sick**

2 An acute illness is a **short-term** illness that can be mild or severe.

3 A chronic illness is a **long-term** illness that can be mild or severe.

4 Following a convulsion, the child needs to be placed in the recovery position, that is, **lying on the side** to prevent the airway to the lungs from becoming blocked by the tongue or by vomit.

5 The tonsils normally enlarge after the age of **5 years and shrink after the age of 10**. Removal only needs to be considered if there are frequent bouts of tonsillitis that cannot be prevented by medicines.

6 Children with diarrhoea are liable to become **dehydrated** (short of water) and should be given plenty to drink.

7 A child with a fever should **be allowed to cool off** to reduce the temperature, for example by sponging with tepid water and lowering the heating in the room.

Total number of marks   18
First time score   ....
Score after revision   ....

1 A medical word that ends in 'itis' indicates that there is swelling in a part of the body often, but not always, due to infection. Place the names of these illnesses against the part of the body which is affected.

appendicitis
arthritis
bronchitis
conjunctivitis
dermatitis

gastritis
hepatitis
laryngitis
meningitis
tonsillitis

.... x

.... ix

....viii

.... vii

.... vi

i...

ii...

iii...

iv...

v...

2 Dean was feeling unwell and complaining of feeling hot and sick, was coughing a lot and didn't want anything to eat. His mother didn't think there was any reason to call a doctor because he was not in much pain and didn't have difficulty in breathing, but sat quietly watching his favourite video.

Why did Dean's mum know that he was not well?

i ....

ii ....

iii ....

iv ....

Why did she decide not to call the doctor?

v ....

vi ....

vii ....

3 Baby Gemma was fretful and showed little interest in anything and her parents realised that she was not very well. She then developed a fever, was sick and had a convulsion. Her parents decided that it was time to contact a doctor.

Why did Gemma's parents know that she was not very well?

i ....

ii ....

What changes took place in Gemma's condition that required a medical opinion?

iii ....

iv ....

v ....

4 It is unusual for babies who are unwell to:
A have a temperature
B be fretful
C be difficult to please
D have convulsions

5 Which disease needs urgent medical attention?
A rubella
B common cold
C chicken pox
D meningitis

1   i   **meningitis**
     ii   **conjunctivitis**
     iii   **bronchitis**
     iv   **dermatitis**
     v   **gastritis**
     vi   **arthritis**
     vii   **appendicitis**
     viii **hepatitis**
     ix   **laryngitis**
     x   **tonsillitis**

2   Dean's mother knew that he was not well because he:
     i   **was feeling hot**
     ii   **was feeling sick**
     iii   **was coughing a lot**
     iv   **didn't want anything to eat**

     She decided not to call the doctor because he:
     v   **was not in much pain**
     vi   **did not have difficulty in breathing**
     vii   **was content to watch a video**

3   Gemma's parents knew that she was not well because she:
     i   **was fretful**
     ii   **showed little interest in anything**

     They decided to contact a doctor when she:
     iii   **developed a fever**
     vi   **was sick**
     v   **had a convulsion**

4   It is quite common for babies who are feeling unwell to have a temperature, be fretful and difficult to please. But it is unusual for them to **have convulsions**.

5   **Meningitis** needs urgent medical attention.

Total number of marks	24
First time score	....
Score after revision	....

Complete this wordsearch by finding all the words in the box below. The words can be forwards, backwards, horizontal, vertical or diagonal.

fever	appetite	headache
health	hospital	diarrhoea
illness	vomiting	quarantine
poison	asthma	convulsion
allergy	antibiotic	cleanliness
eczema	medicine	temperature

C	T	E	M	P	E	R	A	T	U	R	E	T	H	D	D
L	E	C	Z	H	F	I	L	L	E	C	T	A	U	Q	I
E	M	Z	I	A	E	L	L	M	L	J	O	F	T	U	A
A	F	E	V	E	R	C	O	T	E	E	G	M	E	H	R
N	C	M	E	D	I	C	I	N	E	R	R	A	A	E	R
L	G	A	A	D	Q	U	E	N	B	O	G	G	O	A	H
I	H	L	D	P	M	C	G	O	T	N	S	Y	Y	D	O
N	A	C	O	N	V	U	L	S	I	O	N	H	C	A	E
E	I	B	O	N	E	Z	Y	T	G	E	N	C	M	C	A
S	L	C	H	O	S	P	I	T	A	L	F	N	E	H	L
S	L	N	D	G	E	M	O	E	S	S	I	O	T	E	X
B	N	O	S	I	O	P	A	C	K	H	T	L	A	E	H
R	E	D	E	V	F	H	A	B	M	E	S	H	I	O	V
E	S	G	C	I	A	P	P	E	T	I	T	E	M	A	Z
M	S	Q	U	A	R	A	N	T	I	N	E	B	F	A	E
C	L	P	A	K	A	N	T	I	B	I	O	T	I	C	D

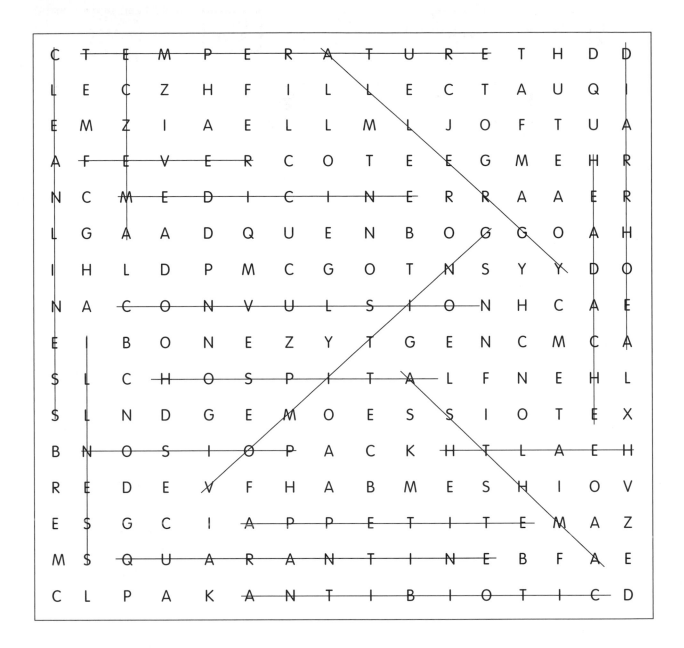

```
C  T  E  M  P  E  R  A  T  U  R  E  T  H  D  D
L  E  C  Z  H  F  I  L  L  E  C  T  A  U  Q  I
E  M  Z  I  A  E  L  L  M  L  J  O  F  T  U  A
A  F  E  V  E  R  C  O  T  E  E  G  M  E  H  R
N  C  M  E  D  I  C  I  N  E  R  R  A  A  E  R
L  G  A  A  D  Q  U  E  N  B  O  G  G  O  A  H
I  H  L  D  P  M  C  G  O  T  N  S  Y  Y  D  O
N  A  C  O  N  V  U  L  S  I  O  N  H  C  A  E
E  I  B  O  N  E  Z  Y  T  G  E  N  C  M  C  A
S  L  C  H  O  S  P  I  T  A  L  F  N  E  H  L
S  L  N  D  G  E  M  O  E  S  S  I  O  T  E  X
B  N  O  S  I  O  P  A  C  K  H  T  L  A  E  H
R  E  D  E  V  F  H  A  B  M  E  S  H  I  O  V
E  S  G  C  I  A  P  P  E  T  I  T  E  M  A  Z
M  S  Q  U  A  R  A  N  T  I  N  E  B  F  A  E
C  L  P  A  K  A  N  T  I  B  I  O  T  I  C  D
```

Total number of marks   18
First time score   ....
Score after revision   ....

1 To help reduce the risk of accidents, many goods are labelled to show that they have been approved for safety. Identify each of the labels above by drawing a sketch in the appropriate box

made to the correct British Standard		harmful or irritant substance		fire resistant	
complies with European regulations		corrosive substance		slow to burn	
meets regulations for domestic electrical appliances		toxic/very toxic		a fire risk	

2 Accidents to children are classified in various categories, for example categories i–x below. Place each of the injuries listed here in its appropriate category.

bead in the nostril
greenstick fracture
black eye
scalded with hot liquid

loss of consciousness
scratches
bleach in the eye

sprained ankle
cut hand
swallowing a pin

i   superficial injury ....

ii   open wound ....

iii   burn ....

iv   bruise ....

v   concussion ....

vi   bone injury ....

vii   joint/tendon injury ....

viii   chemical injury ....

ix   non-injurious foreign body ....

x   injurious foreign body ....

1 Labels that to help prevent accidents:

made to the correct British Standard

harmful or irritant substance

fire resistant

complies with European regulations

corrosive substance

slow to burn

meets regulations for domestic electrical appliances

toxic/very toxic

a fire risk

2 Accident categories:

i	superficial injury	**scratches**
ii	open wound	**cut hand**
iii	burn	**scalded with hot liquid**
iv	bruise	**black eye**
v	concussion	**loss of consciousness**
vi	bone injury	**greenstick fracture**
vii	joint/tendon injury	**sprained ankle**
viii	chemical injury	**bleach in the eye**
ix	non-injurious foreign body	**bead in the nostril**
x	injurious foreign body	**swallowing a pin**

Total number of marks   19
First time score   ....
Score after revision   ....

Non-fatal accidents in the home (national estimates in 000s)		
Type of accident	0–4 years	5–14 years
Falls	230	142
Struck by an object	111	115
Foreign body	36	16
Poisoning	32	4
Heat/fire	31	12
Cut/tear/puncture	26	44
Pinch/crush	25	20

Fatal accidents in the home		
Type of accident	0–4 years	5–14 years
Fires	47	25
Drowning	18	2
Choking/suffocation	14	9
Falls	8	6
Hot substances	6	1
Poisoning	3	2
Electrical	0	0

Source: Home Accident Data Base

Answer questions 1–6 using the data in the tables above.

1 Which accident occurs most often to children in the home?..

2 Name the two non-fatal accidents that occur in similar numbers in both age groups:

i ....

ii ....

3 Apart from falls, being struck by an object, and pinch/crush, name the other causes of non-fatal accidents:

....

....

4 Name the three different ways in which heat-related accidents are classified in the tables above:

i ....

ii ....

iii ....

5 Name the four causes of fatal accidents that are not listed in the causes of non-fatal accidents:

i ....

ii ....

iii ....

iv ....

6 Name the fatal accident which is:

i nine times more common in younger children than older ones......................................

ii 50% more common in younger children than older ones...

1 **Falls** are the most common type of accident that occurs to children in the home.

2 The non-fatal accidents which occur in similar numbers in both age groups are:
being struck by an object
pinch/crush.

3 Apart from falls, being struck by an object, and pinch/crush, the other causes of non-fatal accidents are:
foreign body, e.g. a bead stuck in the ear
poisoning
heat/fire
cut/tear/puncture.

4 The three different ways in which heat-related accidents are classified in the tables are:
heat/fire
fires
hot substances.

5 The four causes of fatal accidents that are not listed in the causes of non-fatal accidents are:
drowning
choking/suffocation
hot substances
electrical.

6 i Being killed by **drowning** is nine times (18:2) more common in younger children than older ones.
   ii Being killed by **poisoning** is 50% (3:2) more common in younger children than older ones.

Total number of marks	16
First time score	....
Score after revision	....

1 Immunisation will protect children with cuts or scratches from catching:
A tetanus
B hepatitis
C meningitis
D tuberculosis

2 Babies and small children can drown in less than:
A 3 cm of water
B 5 cm of water
C 10 cm of water
D 15 cm of water

3 Babies in cars are safer when they travel:
A on the back seat of a car
B on the lap of an adult
C in a child seat
D in a baby carrier strapped to a car seat

4 The person responsible for seeing that a child wears a seat belt is the:
A driver
B parent
C child
D car owner

Child Road Casualties in Great Britain, 2001				
	Killed	Serious injury	Slight injury	Total
Pedestrians 0–4	16	300	1383	1699
5–7	16	529	2063	
Cyclists 0–4	1	7	73	
5–7	2	64	554	
Car passengers 0–4	18	167	2824	
5–7	10	104	2384	
Bus/coach passengers 0–4	0	14	374	
5–7	0	4	465	
Total				
Source: Road Accidents in Gt Britain: 2001 The Casualty Report				

Using the table above:
5 i Add up the columns across to find the number of children killed or injured in each age group.

ii Add up the columns lengthways to find the total number of children killed, seriously injured and slightly injured.

iii How many children under the age of eight years were killed in 2001?   ....

iv How many children were killed or injured in 2001?   ....

6 The number of children of all ages killed was greatest for:
A pedestrians
B cyclists
C car passengers
D bus/coach passengers

7 More children were road casualties in the age group 0–4 than in the age group 5–7 as:
A pedestrians
B cyclists
C car passengers
D bus/coach passengers

1 Children will be protected from **tetanus** if they have been immunised against it. Tetanus germs exist in soil and dirt and enter the body through cuts and scratches.

2 Babies and small children can drown in less than **3 cm of water**.

3 Babies in cars are safer when they travel **in a baby carrier strapped to a car seat**.

4 The person responsible for seeing that a child wears a seat belt is the **driver**.

Child Road Casualties in Great Britain, 2001				
	Killed	Serious injury	Slight injury	Total
Pedestrians				
0–4	16	300	1383	**1699**
5–7	16	529	2063	**2608**
Cyclists				
0–4	1	7	73	**81**
5–7	2	64	554	**620**
Car passengers				
0–4	18	167	2824	**3009**
5–7	10	104	2384	**2498**
Bus/coach passengers				
0–4	0	14	374	**388**
5–7	0	4	465	**469**
Total	63	1189	10120	11372

5 i See **right-hand column** in the table above.
   ii See **bottom row** in the table above.
   iii **63** children under the age of eight years were killed in 2001.
   iv **11372** children were killed or injured in 2001.

6 The number of children of all ages killed was greatest for **pedestrians**.

7 More children were road casualties in the age group 0–4 than in the age group 5–7 as **car passengers**.

Total number of marks	19
First time score	....
Score after revision	....

Across

1 Stand here while waiting to cross a road (4)

3 Part of a car in which a child's fingers can be trapped when it is being closed (4)

6 This is heavy along busy roads (7)

7 A call for help or rescue (3)

8 Cyclists should not do this on a pavement (4)

9 Vehicles that are bigger than bicycles but smaller than buses (4)

11 When in traffic, cyclists should ride in __ __ __ __ le file (6)

13 Look and __ __ __ __ __ __ before crossing the road (6)

15 Young children are not good judges of the __ __ __ __ __ at which vehicles are travelling

16 Children need to be taught how to __ __ __ __ __ __ busy roads (5)

Down

1 This type of mark on baby carriers shows that they have been made to the correct British Standard (4)

2 The Green Cross Code teaches children about __ __ __ __ safety (4)

3 These people are responsible for seeing that children under 14 are either in child seats or are wearing seat belts (6)

4 A boy is __ __ __ __ __ __ __ his life if he runs into a busy road after a ball (7)

5 Risk of an accident increases if this person distracts the car driver (9)

9 __ __ __ __ __ __ need to be the right size for comfort and safety (6)

10 __ __ __ __ belts should always be used (4)

12 When are bicycles allowed to be ridden without lights at night-time? (5)

14 A small child cannot __ __ __ over parked cars (3)

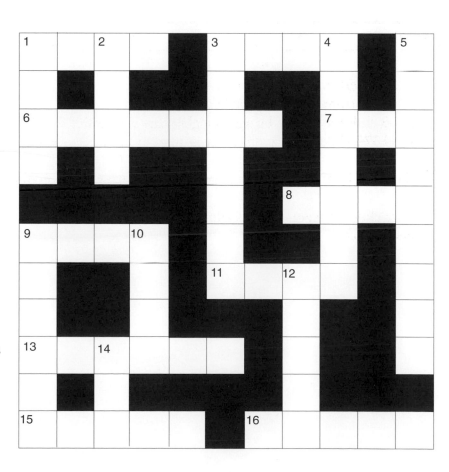

Crossword grid (answers):

Across / Down letters:

- Row 1: K(1) E R B(2) — D(3) O O R(4) — P(5)
- Row 2: I — O — R — I — A
- Row 3: T(6) R A F F I C — S(7) O S
- Row 4: E — D — V — K — S
- Row 5: — — — E — R(8) I D E
- Row 6: C(9) A R S(10) — R — N — N
- Row 7: Y — E — S(11) I N(12) G — G
- Row 8: C — A — E — E
- Row 9: L(13) I S(14) T E N — V — R
- Row 10: E — E — E
- Row 11: S(15) P E E D — C(16) R O S S

Total number of marks	19
First time score	....
Score after revision	....

SECTION 8 THE FAMILY AND THE COMMUNITY

CONTENTS

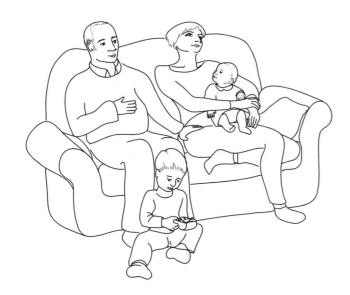

Celia lives with her husband Simon and two children, Mark who is 6 years old, and Gemma who has just had her first birthday. She decided that she wanted to return to her old job for three days a week but first she had to make sure that the children were cared for while she was at work. So Celia started to ask questions.

Answer the questions below.

	Yes/No
1 Do childminders take children as young as Gemma?	
2 Is Mark too old to be cared for by a childminder?	
3 Do childminders always have to be registered?	
4 If the children are looked after by their grandmother, does she have to be registered?	
5 Can a friend act as a childminder without registering?	
6 Should a childminder care for more than three children under the age of five?	
7 Does this maximum number include the childminder's own children?	
8 Are childminders expected to look after children who are ill?	
9 Are childminders' homes inspected for safety and cleanliness?	
10 Are nannies required to be registered with the Local Authority or OFSTED?	
11 Do all nannies have a qualification in child care?	
12 Do all mother's helps have a qualification in child care?	
13 Do day nurseries provide all-day care?	
14 Do children at day nurseries have to attend every day?	
15 Do children at day nurseries have to attend for the whole day?	
16 Do any crèches provide all-day care?	
17 Do all out-of-school care schemes offer care only at the end of the school day?	
18 Would Gemma be able to attend a holiday care scheme if necessary?	

1 Yes.

2 No. Generally, childminders care for children under the age of 8 years.

3 Yes. Childminders have to be registered and regularly inspected by OFSTED (Office for Standards in Education).

4 No. Close relatives can act as childminders without being registered.

5 No. The friend would be breaking the law.

6 No. Three is the maximum number of children under five that a childminder can care for.

7 Yes.

8 No. Children who are ill need much attention, and may be infectious.

9 Yes. Childminders' homes are inspected once a year.

10 No.

11 No.

12 No.

13 Yes.

14 No. Children attend on a regular basis, one or more times a week.

15 No. They can attend for the full day or part of the day.

16 Yes. Some provide all-day care, for example those run by hospitals and businesses.

17 No. Some out-of-school care schemes offer care before school starts.

18 No. Holiday care schemes are for school-aged children.

Total number of marks   18
First time score   ....
Score after revision   ....

Complete these words by searching for the answers in the wordsearch below.

i   The Local Authority department in charge of children in care:

S __ __ __ __ __   S __ __ __ __ __ __ __

ii   The Act of Parliament, 1989, concerned with children in care:

C __ __ __ __ __ __ __   A __ __

iii This compels parents to hand over their child to be looked

after by others: C __ __ __ __   O __ __ __ __

iv   The type of agreement when parents agree for their children

to be in care: V __ __ __ __ __ __ __ __

v   An arrangement for children to live in other people's home:

F __ __ __ __ __ __ __ __

vi   A legal process by which adults become parents of other

people's children: A __ __ __ __ __ __ __

vii The time before a child becomes legally part of a new

family is called a: P __ __ __ __ __ __ __ __ __ __ __   P __ __ __ __ __

A	S	O	C	I	A	L	O	B	I	N	E	S	D
W	E	S	C	H	F	I	C	O	A	O	L	P	F
P	R	O	B	A	T	I	O	N	A	R	Y	S	O
E	V	R	E	P	O	Q	U	N	E	A	L	C	S
R	I	E	D	I	N	O	R	D	E	R	S	R	T
I	C	C	A	G	N	E	T	E	A	M	T	H	E
O	E	S	H	A	D	E	N	X	Y	M	E	B	R
D	S	W	O	P	R	I	S	E	N	I	A	L	I
A	S	H	A	O	K	C	H	I	L	D	R	E	N
J	A	D	O	P	T	I	O	N	G	E	N	I	G
N	E	B	A	C	E	X	Y	T	H	S	A	C	T
R	I	D	E	I	V	F	S	M	O	E	S	O	N
P	E	R	V	O	L	U	N	T	A	R	Y	O	L
C	L	O	U	R	W	T	I	V	I	S	O	F	E

i   **SOCIAL SERVICES**

ii   **CHILDREN ACT**

iii **COURT ORDER**

iv   **VOLUNTARY**

v   **FOSTERING**

vi   **ADOPTION**

vii **PROBATIONARY PERIOD**

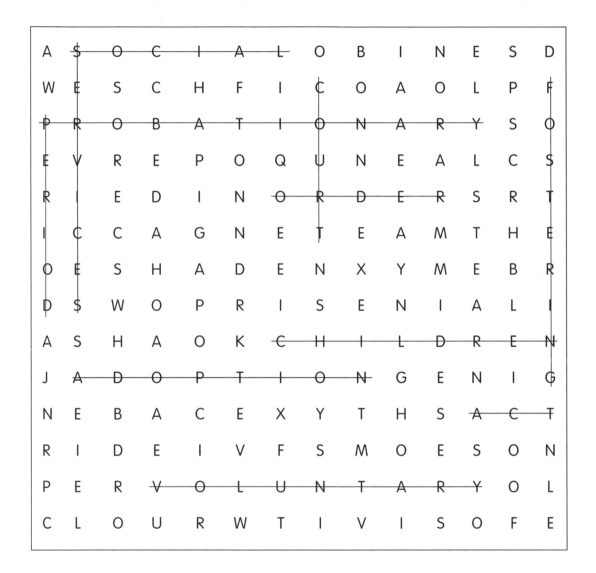

Total number of marks   11
First time score   ....
Score after revision   ....

1 A congenital abnormality is:
A delayed development
B present at birth
C malfunctioning of the sex organs
D a sensory disability

2 Down's syndrome results from:
A a learning difficulty
B delayed development
C a sensory disability
D a chromosome disorder

3 Deafness is:
A a physical disability
B a learning disability
C a sensory disability
D a social disability

4 Muscular dystrophy is:
A a physical disability
B a learning disability
C a sensory disability
D a social disability

5 Autism is a:
A a physical disability
B a learning disability
C a sensory disability
D a social disability

6 Cerebral palsy results from:
A an abnormal gene
B lack of interest in other people
C slow growth
D brain damage at birth

7 Asperger's syndrome results in:
A an abnormal gene
B a lack of social understanding
C slow growth
D brain damage at birth

8 Haemophilia results from:
A an abnormal gene
B a lack of social understanding
C slow growth
D brain damage at birth

9 A child's peers are:
A adults who are in charge
B adults in the family
C other children in the family
D other children of the same age group

10 Skills for daily living are the speciality of:
A physiotherapists
B occupational therapists
C language therapists
D SEN specialists

11 Speech problems are the speciality of:
A physiotherapists
B occupational therapists
C language therapists
D SEN specialists

12 Mobility difficulties are the speciality of:
A physiotherapists
B occupational therapists
C language therapists
D SEN specialists

13 Advice on education is the speciality of:
A physiotherapists
B occupational therapists
C language therapists
D SEN specialists

14 A national society for people with autism is:
A ASBAH
B NAS
C SCOPE
D ICAN

15 An association for people with spina bifida is:
A ASBAH
B NAS
C SCOPE
D ICAN

16 An organisation for people with cerebral palsy is:
A ASBAH
B NAS
C SCOPE
D ICAN

1 A congenital abnormality is a disability **present at birth**.

2 Down's syndrome results from **a chromosome disorder**.

3 Deafness is **a sensory disability**.

4 Muscular dystrophy is **a physical disability**.

5 Autism is **a social disability**.

6 Cerebral palsy results from **brain damage at birth**.

7 Asperger's syndrome results in **lack of social understanding**.

8 Haemophilia results from **an abnormal gene**.

9 A child's peers are **other children of the same age group**.

10 Skills for daily living are the concern of **occupational therapists**.

11 Speech problems are the concern of **language therapists**.

12 Mobility difficulties are the concern of **physiotherapists**.

13 Advice on education is the concern of **SEN specialists** (SEN = Special Educational Needs).

14 A national society for people with autism is **NAS** (NAS = National Autistic Society).

15 An association for people with spina bifida is **ASBAH** (ASBAH = Association for Spina Bifida and Hydrocephalus).

16 An organisation for people with cerebral palsy is **SCOPE**.

Total number of marks	16
First time score	....
Score after revision	....

1 Which organisation checks children's eyesight?
A Social Security
B National Health Service
C Social Services
D Local Authority (the Council)

2 Which organisation gives financial help (cash)?
A Benefits Agency
B National Health Service
C Social Services
D Local Authority (the Council)

3 Which organisation gives housing benefit?
A Benefits Agency
B National Health Service
C Social Services
D Local Authority (the Council)

4 Which organisation supervises children in care?
A Social Security
B National Health Service
C Social Services
D Local Authority (the Council)

5 Which organisation supports families with special needs?
A Social Security
B National Health Service
C Social Services
D Local Authority (the Council)

6 Which organisation has adoption services?
A Social Security
B National Health Service
C Social Services
D Local Authority (the Council)

7 Which organisation provides family planning advice?
A Social Security
B National Health Service
C Social Services
D Local Authority (the Council)

8 Which organisation provides free dental checks during pregnancy?
A Social Security
B National Health Service
C Social Services
D Local Authority (the Council)

9 Child Benefit is paid to the:
A child
B child or parent
C child or guardian
D person with whom the child lives

10 Maternity Pay is a benefit for:
A working women before the birth
B women not in employment
C working women before and after the birth
D working women after they have given birth

11 Match each voluntary organisation with its function (clues are underlined).

Voluntary organisation	Function
i CHILDREN 1st (RSSPCC)	for the prevention of cruelty to children
ii CGF	raises funds for a better world for children
iii CPAG	gives advice on children's growth problems
iv Kidscape	for the welfare of Scottish children
v NSPCC	campaigns against bullying and child abuse
vi SCF	acts for relief of poverty amongst children

1 Checking children's eyesight is the responsibility of the **National Health Service**.

2 Financial help (cash) is given by the **Benefits Agency**.

3 Housing benefit is given by the **Local Authority (the Council)**.

4 Children in care are supervised by the **Social Services**.

5 **Social Services** support families with special needs.

6 **Adoption services** are provided by the Social Services.

7 The **National Health Service** provides family planning advice.

8 The **National Health Service** provides free dental checks during pregnancy.

9 Child Benefit is paid to the **person with whom the child lives**.

10 Maternity pay is a benefit for **working women before and after the birth**.

11 i   CHILDREN 1st (RSSPCC) – **for the welfare of Scottish children** (Royal Scottish Society for the Prevention of Cruelty to Children)

ii   CGF – **gives advice on children's growth problems** (Child Growth Foundation)

iii   CPAG – **acts for relief of poverty amongst children** (Child Poverty Action Group)

iv   Kidscape – **campaigns against bullying and child abuse**

v   NSPCC – **for the prevention of cruelty to children** (National Society for the Prevention of Cruelty to Children)

vi   SCF – **raises funds for a better world for children** (Save the Children Fund)

Total number of marks	16
First time score	....
Score after revision	....

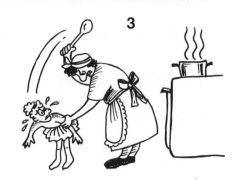

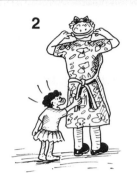

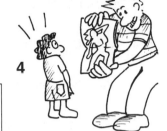

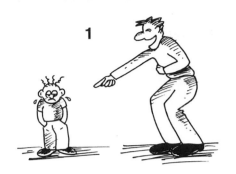

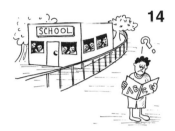

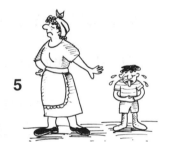

Ways in which children are abused

Match each picture with its description.

		Number
i	Hitting or hurting	
ii	Breaking down self-confidence	
iii	Leaving a child without supervision	
iv	Not listening to a child	
v	Teasing a child unnecessarily	
vi	Forcing a child to touch you	
vii	Bribing a child to keep quiet	
viii	Verbally abusing a child	
ix	Exposing a child to pornography	
x	Neglecting a child's medical needs	
xi	Not taking proper care of a child	
xii	Showing no affection to a child	
xiii	Neglecting a child's educational needs	
xiv	Touching where a child doesn't want to be touched	

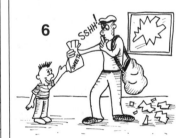

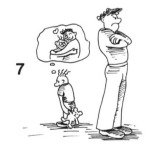

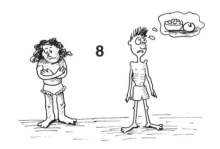

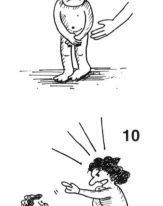

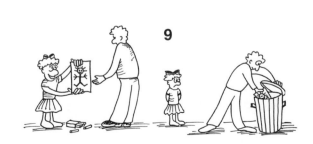

Adapted from the poster 'What is Child Abuse', available from Smallwood Publishing Ltd, The Old Bakery, Charlton House, Dour Street, Dover, Kent CT16 1ED   tel. 01304 226800   email info@smallwood.co.uk

Ways in which children are abused:

		Number
i	Hitting or hurting	3
ii	Breaking down self-confidence	9
iii	Leaving a child without supervision	12
iv	Not listening to a child	2
v	Teasing a child unnecessarily	1
vi	Forcing a child to touch you	13
vii	Bribing a child to keep quiet	6
viii	Verbally abusing a child	10
ix	Exposing a child to pornography	4
x	Neglecting a child's medical needs	5
xi	Not taking proper care of a child	8
xii	Showing no affection to a child	7
xiii	Neglecting a child's educational needs	14
xiv	Touching where a child doesn't want to be touched	11

Total number of marks	14
First time score	....
Score after revision	....

True/false

1   Marriage is a legal contract between two people

2   Co-habitation means living together without going through a marriage ceremony

3. Co-habitation gives the couple the same legal rights as marriage

4   Reconciliation is an attempt to restore a marriage

5   RELATE is only concerned with relationships between parents and children

6   RELATE gives marriage guidance advice

7   The Children Act 1989 covers most aspects of law relating to children

8   Parental responsibilities are those duties decided by the parents

9   Parental responsibilities are legal requirements

10 In court cases involving children, the welfare of the child is the most important factor

11 In court cases involving children, the views of the parents are the most important factor

12 In court cases, children take part in decisions about their future

13 Parents only have legal responsibility if their children live with them

14 Parents have legal responsibility if their children do not live with them

15 Parents are responsible for their children's attendance at school

16 Parents are not legally responsible for their child's actions outside the home

17 An official Guardian can be appointed by parents while they go on holiday

18 When a child is left without parents, an official guardian is appointed

19 Divorce occurs when a marriage has broken down

20 Divorce is the legal ending of a marriage

21 Child Maintenance is money paid by Social Security for the upkeep of children

22 Child Maintenance is administered by the Child Support Agency

1 True.

2 True.

3 False.

4 True.

5 False. RELATE (formerly called The Marriage Guidance Council) counsels on all aspects of family relationships including marriage guidance.

6 True.

7 True.

8 False. Parental responsibilities are defined by law as all the rights, duties, powers and authority which by law a parent of a child has in relation to the child and his property.

9 True.

10 True.

11 False. In courts cases, the welfare of the child is of utmost importance.

12 True.

13. False.

14 True.

15 True.

16 False.

17 False. Official Guardians are appointed for children without parents, i.e. the parents have died.

18 True.

19 False. A marriage which has broken down need not be followed by divorce.

20 True.

21 False. Child Maintenance is paid by non-resident parents towards the upkeep of their child.

22 True.

Total number of marks	22
First time score	....
Score after revision	....